A SEARCH FOR WELLNESS

(non-fiction)

by F. KANSAS MATTSON

Dear Robert
Here is to your good health
Best wishes
Frank Kansas Mattson
Dec 15 1990

A SEARCH FOR WELLNESS
How to Turn Back Your Biological Clock

By F. Kansas Mattson

Published by:

SUPER G Publishing Company
Post Office Box 7560
Hampton, Virginia 23666

First printing 1990
Printed in Fredericksburg, Virginia, U.S.A.

Library of Congress Cataloging in Publication Data
Library of Congress Number 90–70585
Mattson, Frank K.
A Search for Wellness: How to Turn Back Your
  Biological Clock
F. Kansas Mattson.—first edition
Bibliography: p.
Includes index.

ISBN 0–9625584–7–8: $16.95 Hardcover

DEDICATION

To the men and women who take personal responsibility for the maintenance of their health.

EPIGRAPH

Thy food shall be thy remedy. Nature heals, the physician is only nature's assistant.

Hippocrates
Father of Medicine
circa 400 B.C.

The doctor of the future will give no medicine but will interest his patients in the care of the human frame, in diet, and in the cause and prevention of disease.

Thomas A. Edison
1847–1941

NOTICE

This book is one man's story of a search for wellness. It is not intended to be a blueprint for the reader to follow, in part or whole. Try the therapies in this book only with the advice and guidance of your personal physician and other health professionals.

TABLE OF CONTENTS

FOREWORD

After being told repeatedly by his physician that there was no cure for many of his illnesses, and that he would have to learn to live with them, Mr. Mattson decided to take personal responsibility for his health, and sought physicians and therapists who would work with him to find both causes and cures.

The book is not a prescription—but describes techniques that can be used by anyone to find a physician/therapist who will work with them to feel better, look younger, reduce their biological age, and in many cases cure "incurable" illnesses. The author makes several key points throughout the book. First, make a decision to get well. Second, take personal responsibility for your health, and eliminate lifestyle factors that may be contributing to your condition like inadequate exercise, poor diet, cigarette smoking, or excess consumption of alcohol. Third, find a physician/therapist who is willing to work with you to find answers to your own health problems. Finally, no single therapist may have all the answers, and a treatment that works for one person may not work for another. Therefore, it is necessary to judiciously select therapeutic regimens that work for you. Mr. Mattson found that a combination of therapies by medical doctors, chiropractors, dentists, and nutritionists were required to restore his health.

Mr. Mattson suggests several books and newsletters that will serve as excellent starting points in a search for wellness. Names of medical doctors who are knowledgeable of many of the alternative therapies (both medical and non-medical) which he describes in the book may be found by contacting the American College of Advancement in Medicine (714) 583-7666, as mentioned in the book.

I highly recommend this book to anyone who has been told by their physician that "there is no cure, and you'll have to learn to live with it". There *may* be a cure, and you *may* not have to live with your pain and discomfort.

Ward Dean, M.D.
Medical Director
The Center for Bio-Gerontology
Pensacola, FL

Author, *Biological Aging Measurement—Clinical Applications*

PREFACE

This book, *A Search for Wellness,* addresses a number of experiences relating to the restoration and/or maintenance of my health at an optimum level. I found the notion of "aging diseases" to be largely a myth. Many of the infirming conditions people call "inevitable" do not have to happen. Probably the most exciting endeavor for people above age forty is to get educated and practice personal behaviors that result in good health. I say "above age forty" because that is about the time one's health begins to slip. Success will come with a change in living habits.

Life is a game and the outcome depends to a great extent on how you follow the rules. You are what you eat, and you become what you think about most. Either you are in control of your health, or you are out of control, drifting through life.

Imagine buying a fine, expensive automobile
—giving it no "TLC"—much less the specified maintenance
—using cheap gas
—using cheap oil; not changing the filter
—running on underinflated tires
Is that smart?—How will this car perform?

In like manner, many humans insult their bodies by
—smoking
—drinking to excess
—eating excessively (especially food containing fat, sugar and caffeine)
—not exercising
—taking unnecessary risks

Is this smart? How long do you think these individuals will live. How do you think they'll feel as long as they do live? Do you think they'll "*live* until they die?" When you get your priorities straight and take care of your health, the rest of the activities you indulge in become more pleasant and fruitful.

I used to have the attitude I could do anything I wanted without worrying about my health so long as I continued to function and didn't have too many stomachaches or headaches. I tended to consign health maintenance to the doctor, just like I take my car to the mechanic when it breaks down. Many times I knew the cause of my sickness even before I saw the doctor—I needed to change my habits!

This book is a story of a search for wellness—my personal experience with declining health, and the remarkable turnaround after taking charge and accepting responsibility. This is one of the most exciting challenges of my lifetime. I made health maintenance priority number one. In the last six years, I reshaped my physical appearance, improved my health, and increased my energy level. In the process, I discovered a number of legitimate alternative treatments/therapies that don't seem to be widely known.

It is my ambition and hope that *A Search for Wellness* will bring a new awareness regarding health maintenance to the public. Taking personal responsibility can lead to a more fruitful and enjoyable life.

CHAPTER 1

The Challenge

My name is Kansas and I am an Aquarius. About the time I decided to write this book I spotted this horoscope: "*Aquarius*—Your theories are under fire from all sides. Little is gained by an immediate defense. Renewed resolution comes later. Consider how to improve your health." So, I gave serious attention to this subject which turned out to be an interesting adventure.

My doctor declared there is no known cure for my sudden affliction with a dry mouth and dry eyes. He got my attention when he said my symptoms were a typical forerunner of collagen vascular disease which involves stiffening of joints and multiple organ failure. The challenge became clear—find the cure! In the process not only did I overcome my dry mouth and dry eyes, but I overcame many things I thought to be normal aging diseases.

My story starts when I reached age 60, but of course I reflect on an earlier time as I discuss the physical profile of my health. This is an account of treating the cause to correct problems, as opposed to treating the symptoms. It is a story of success.

So who am I? I was a Monday child born on "Kansas Day," January 29, 1923 in Glenn Ellyn, a suburb of Chicago, but my roots come from Kansas. The birthing happened at home with a doctor and practical nurse in attendance. I weighed in at 10$^{1}/_{2}$ pounds, the biggest from a brood of five boys; and breast fed (this information courtesy of my 96-year-old mother).

In January 1923, political turmoil abounded. The Turks were at war. A revolutionary war was in progress in China. France and Germany were having it out over Alsace-Lorraine. President Harding refused to get involved. You could get gas at most places for 15 cents a gallon or less. At the Hotel Rittenhouse, which catered to the best patronage, in Philadelphia, a room with bath came at $3.00. The hotel served dinner for $1.25. Charlie Chaplin announced his engagement to Pola Negri. These were momentous times!

I grew up in the state of Kansas. One year after graduating from Topeka High School, I joined the Army. I soon found myself in India as a pilot flying cargo over the "Hump," the India-to-China route during World War II. Not too long after returning from India, I got married and had two sons. My family shared the major portion of twenty-one years of military service, which included about thirty different stations. During this time I got my college education through night school. After leaving the military service, I joined a major aerospace company and worked in a field marketing office. As I write this, I am nearing my twenty-fifth anniversary with my company.

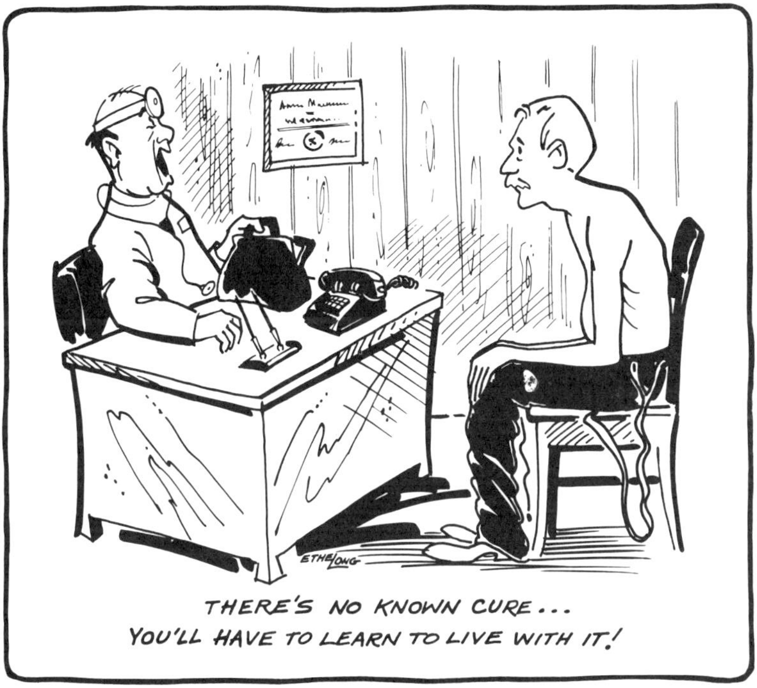
ETHELONG
THERE'S NO KNOWN CURE...
YOU'LL HAVE TO LEARN TO LIVE WITH IT!

I started off addressing my health problems from a nutritional point of view. This included the understanding of food allergies and the part they play in the struggle to maintain health. Initially I achieved remarkable success but backslid after two years. As I became a bona fide health nut, I soon found myself learning about:

- exercise as it influences health
- chiropractic therapy
- effects of mercury amalgam (fillings) for teeth
- chelation therapy for cardiovascular problems, and removal of toxic metals from the body
- mineral and vitamin supplementation
- malabsorption, a digestive system dysfunction
- macrobiotics, a different dietary regimen
- Hippocrates living food diet and body cleansing program.

The introduction to these many subjects came to me by the way of newsletters from several sources which included:

- *Men's Health*
- Gary Null's *Natural Living Newsletter*
- University of California, *Berkley Wellness Letter*
- *American Institute for Cancer Research Newsletter*
- *Mayo Clinic Health Letter*
- *Nutrition Action Health Letter*, Center for Science in the Public Interest

This is the story of my becoming aware of *eating to live.* In May 1983, I suffered another bout of diverticulitis. Diverticulitis is outpouching in the lower intestine. It becomes sore or inflamed from trapped waste. If this condition persists, there is a danger the colon will become perforated. I reasoned I'd been drinking too much milk (the milk aspect will be explained later). So, I stopped drinking milk, believing the diverticulitis would go away as it had in the past; and it did. But life is full of the unexpected.

About one week later, as my wife and I drove through the countryside on our annual trip to Carlisle, Pa., something happened to me that had never happened before. Suddenly, my mouth went dry to the point of gagging. We stopped to get a drink, but this did little to relieve the condition. Sucking on mints or chewing gum did not help. This first episode lasted about two hours, and remained gone for the rest of the day. However, it returned two or three times the next day and continued to come and go.

I soon learned a lot about the human anatomy, drugs and nutrition. Many of these things I should have learned years earlier.

I learned the human anatomy is a complex chemical factory including an auto-immune system. When the auto-immune system is overwhelmed, temporarily or otherwise, we contract diseases. I also learned saliva generates enzymes as a part of the digestive process. I had thought the saliva just made the food mushy so it could be swallowed easier. Now I understand why my grandmother always told me to chew my food well and not swallow it whole.

I am sure most people know prescription drugs may have side effects. The truth is, they *all* have side effects. Many times these are serious, so a second drug may be administered to dampen the side effects of the first. At times, a chain reaction begins that calls for a third or fourth drug. Soon the human body's own chemical factory becomes thoroughly confused. Meanwhile, some of these drugs may do irreparable damage to one or more organs, glands or a network of nerves, blood vessels and bones that make up the chemical factory.

As I studied the subject of *getting well,* Dr. Henry Beiler and Nathan Pritikin in their respective books convinced me to try nutrition as an alternative to drug treatment. I realized I probably got into trouble from bad nutritional habits and rationalized that the dry eyes and mouth might be corrected by good nutritional habits.

My story, for the most part, is written as it unfolded. Up through Chapter 13 represents the first four years of experience: age 60–64. Then came a one-year lapse in writing, which I picked up with Chapter 14 at age 65. The completion through Chapter 18 came at age 66, which is a six-year time span from the start of my search.

CHAPTER 2

Motivation

I remained *ignorant* about health matters up to age 60, but an awakening came when I developed the affliction of dry mouth and eyes described as incurable. This episode caused me to *think.* Reflecting on the health aspects of my life, I regret this awakening did not occur at an earlier age.

Because of the implications of my dry mouth, I became seriously concerned about my personal health. I believed it to be within my control, but I needed to *think,* and keep on *thinking.* This meant studying, observing, and altering my lifestyle, which involved a goodly amount of detective work.

In reality, I learned many of the health problems classified as *normal aging* should be reclassified. Sure, after years of abuse to your body's chemical factory you will experience a number of dysfunctions. Some of the health problems I include on the list as a result of abuse or improper attention are: diverticulitis, constipation, hemorrhoids, arthritis, bursitis, dry mouth and eyes, weight control problems and cardiovascular disease. By *thinking* and becoming knowledgeable of proper diet and exercise you can reverse many of these so-called aging diseases. If you choose not to adjust your health habits, the accumulation of problems can be overwhelming.

Henry Bieler, MD, author of *Food is Your Best Medicine,* is the person who cleaned the cobwebs from my head and started me *thinking.*

Bieler early on lived the "good life" and soon found himself in trouble with his health. He knew about drugs and the consequences of the side effects and the need to avoid them in his treatment. This set Bieler to *thinking.* His subsequent experience of working with diet changes and without drugs made him believe 80–85 percent of all human ailments are self-limited and run their course in a short time. Most of the time, drugs are not necessary. Early in his book (pages 19–21) he reports the experiences of two seriously ill patients cured by a change in diet.

Dr. Bieler made me aware of putrefaction. My intolerance to beef caused it to rot as it passed through my digestive tract and waste elimination apparatus. I learned the consequences were:

- Putrefaction causes gas with an offensive odor, like sewer gas. Nature tried to tell me something. This does not imply that all foods that you're allergic to putrefy. It pleased me to discover the cause of this difficulty.
- The nutrient value absorbed from food that putrefies as it passes through your system in the digestive process is somewhat diminished.

In understandable language, Bieler explains that the body is a chemical factory.

Bieler presented case histories of patients who recovered from desperate situations. His book, *Food is Your Best Medicine,* motivated me to study, question, investigate, and try different approaches related to regaining and maintaining my health. So far I have read his book from cover to cover four times, an inspiration to change my living habits.

Food is Your Best Medicine got me to *thinking* about a book I had read at least two years earlier, *Pritikin Program for Diet and Exercise* by Nathan Pritikin.

Pritikin in his early 40s learned of his 300 cholesterol count. The master two-step stress test showed some coronary insufficiency. Two years later, another two step test indicated "substantial coronary heart disease."

Pritikin became one of the early pioneers in restoring health by a program of nutrition and exercise. He realized great success in these basic tenets:

- diet—no more than 10 percent of the calories in the daily diet should come from fat. Limit protein to three to four ounces per day. Skip red meat, sugar and white flour.
- exercise—walk, jog, or swim, etc. four or five times per week. Do this for a minimum of 30 minutes to raise your pulse rate.
- zero coffee and other beverages and foods containing caffeine; and no alcohol or tobacco.

A story regarding Pritikin's diet and exercise program comes from Dr. Susan Forward's radio talk show. For those who have not heard of Forward, she is a psychologist considered insightful in her advice to callers. A young lady called one day and explained her problem to Forward. She started dating a handsome man, healthy and financially secure. She

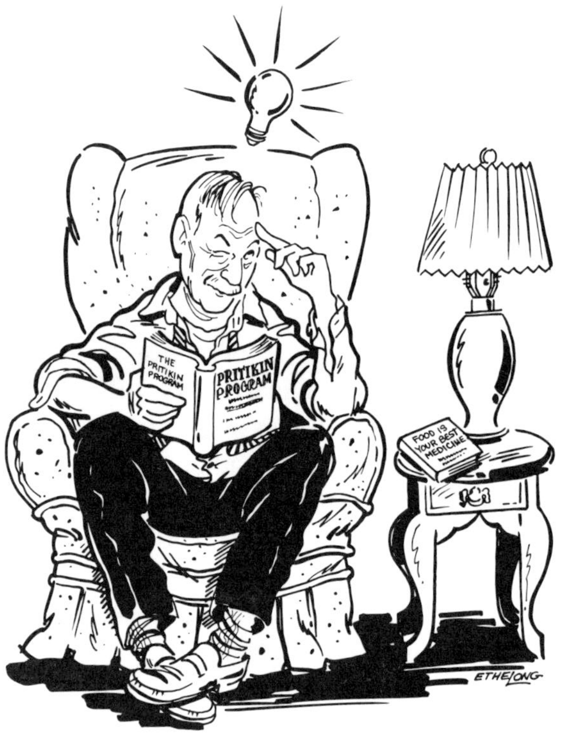

I THINK THERE ARE SOME ANSWERS HERE!

fell in love and wanted to marry this man. This "Pritikin man" refused to marry her unless she took up the Pritikin credo. This young lady did not like the Pritikin program. Forward's response, "Once a Pritikin man, always a Pritikin man; forget it dearie, or join the club." Just to let you know, I am almost a "Pritikin man." My shortcoming is in the fat department; I love nuts. There are about 175 calories in every ounce of walnuts so I sometimes blow the 10 percent rule.

Bieler and Pritikin, my prime motivators, encouraged me to take charge of my own health. I became an avid reader of health books and periodicals. A recent book, *Pass or Bypass,* by James Julian, M.D., reinforced my motivation and conviction.

Some other information made an impression on my *thinking* including three of Gary Null's Natural Living Newsletters (NLN):

- Silver (Mercury Amalgam) Dental Fillings, Newsletter #32.
- Chiropractors, Newsletter Vol. 1, number 5.
- Chelation Part I, Newsletter number 34.
- Chelation Part II, Newsletter number 35.

(These back issues are available NLN Publications, P.O. Box 849, Madison Square Station, New York, NY 10010)

Some other publications influenced me including:

- *Bypassing Bypass* by Elmer Cranton, M.D. and Arline Brecher.
- *Nutrition Against Aging* by Michael A. Weiner, Ph.D. and Kathleen Goss.

Bypassing Bypass's primary thrust deals with chelation therapy to reverse heart disease without surgery. However, Chapter 7 of the book deals with other ailments corrected by chelation therapy including:

- restored vision; reversal of approaching blindness
- reduction of joint stiffness
- recovery of acute symptoms of senility
- lower extremity peripheral vascular problems including gangrene corrected without the benefit of surgical intervention

I found the claims in Chapter 7 of *Bypassing Bypass* confirmed by my own personal observation of fellow patients' experience. These wonderful happenings could be classified as *miracle cures*. Chelation therapy promotes good circulation to all your body parts and eliminates toxic metals from your system at the same time. When the body's natural immune system realizes these benefits, miracles do happen. I address a few miracle stories of my own in Chapter 10.

Nutrition Against Aging reinforced my personal experience that many of the so-called *normal aging diseases* are not necessarily inevitable. Normal aging, to my way of thinking, is misunderstood and/or misrepresented. The cause frequently stems from a nutritional imbalance.

Here is a sample of items from *Nutrition Against Aging* that got my attention:

- *Zinc supplement can control and reverse prostatitis*. It is a gruesome fact that a high percentage of men by the time they reach the age of 60 will have experienced prostate problems. Yet, zinc supplementation to maintain a healthy prostate does not seem to be widely known.
- *Phytates are a danger in bran: phytates interfere with the absorption of zinc, iron and calcium as well as other important mineral nutrients*. This is one among a number of vagaries that relate to nutrition, illustrating the point that moderation in all things is important to good health. It is foolhardy to undertake a health program without the guidance of appropriate and knowledgeable health professionals.
- Chapter Five, "*Speaking of Creaking: Arthritis—The Overlooked Role of Nutrition*", supports fully my personal experience with this "aging disease."

This author addresses a number of diseases which can be affected by nutrition including heart disease, cancer, diabetes, arthritis, senility and serious digestive disorders. This book, *Nutrition Against Aging*, gave me a lot to *think* about.

CHAPTER 3

Health Profile & Transformation

This is the part of my story I enjoy telling. I am fascinated by the physical changes occurring within eighteen months after starting the *search for wellness*. As you will see there are twenty cases of success out of twenty-three chances. First, I will list them chronologically and then go on to discuss each one in detail. Some were a one-time episode; however, the majority were recurring.

1) history of chronic constipation
2) urinary tract disorders
3) continual sinus drainage and stuffy head
4) headaches
5) borderline anemia/chronic fatigue
6) weight control difficulties
7) cold hands and feet
8) prostatic enlargement
9) diverticulitis
10) nocturnal leg and foot cramps
11) cold sores

12) muscles spasms
13) dry nasal passages
14) dry eyes—no tearing action
15) hemorrhoids
16) stomach ulcer
17) brittle nails
18) bursitis
19) arthritis in my finger joints
20) dry mouth—unable to salivate at random times
21) belching and continual passing of foul smelling gas
22) hardening of the arteries
23) cosmetic appearance

Fortunately for me, none of the conditions on this list seemed life-threatening, and I appeared to be in reasonably good shape. After all, I could function and had used only 5 days sick leave in the past 25 years. So, at age 60, I thought (mistakenly) that this was merely a part of the so-called normal aging process. Then, I looked into the subject of nutrition, and when *I made up my mind* to change my diet and eating habits, remarkable transformations followed.

Chronic constipation. The constipation caused hard stools that I managed to move no more than every three to five days.

Before I discovered my food allergy, I took an artificial bulk supplement twice a day for at least five years to alleviate the constipation. Even with artificial bulk, I still experienced waiting three or four days between bowel movements. I considered constipation a part of my normal makeup. However, after discovering my allergy to beef and eliminating beef from my diet, I no longer suffer this aggravation.

Urinary tract disorders. There are two dimensions to be considered. The first is the diminishing force of the stream. I grudgingly admit this may be from aging because my change in health habits has had little effect on this condition. The second is my inability to get through the night without having to get up more than once to go to the bathroom. Now for the second part, since my early youth, a bathroom trip at least

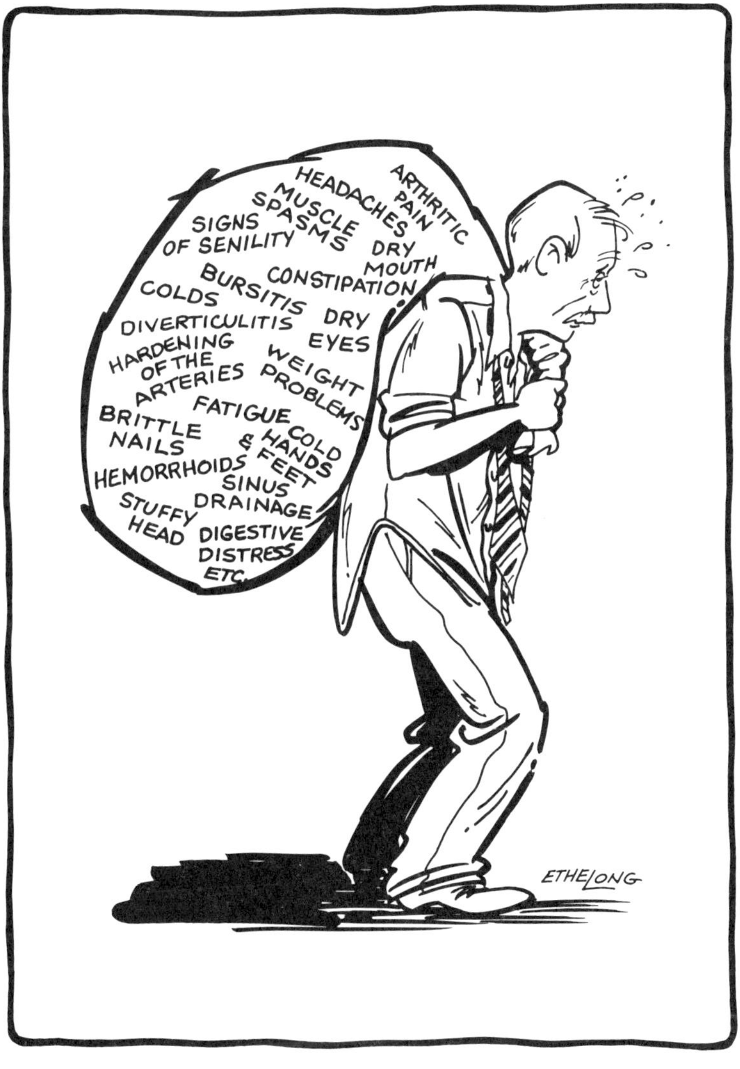

once each night became routine. As the years rolled by this became two, then three, then more.

Over the years, the question always came up during the annual physical, "How many trips do you make to the bathroom at night?" Three or more was a wrong answer. This caused a visit with a urologist. This incurred a bladder inspection on two different occasions with no abnormalities being detected. The instrument used is a fibre optic that allows the doctor to visually inspect the condition of the urinary tract and bladder. Much pain followed in the next two days when I passed water. Years later, after chiropractic spinal manipulation, the problem of frequent visits to the bathroom at night diminished to one trip per night, occasionally none.

Sinus drainage and stuffy head, a long term dysfunction (since age 20) and it has no apparent relationship to a pollen allergy. The sinus drainage was not particularly troublesome, but it did stop up my nose regularly. So I became a mouth breather. My wife chided me to close my mouth and breathe through my nose. "Besides," she said, "you look stupid with your mouth open." As I indicated earlier, 30 days after I stopped drinking milk, my sinus drainage slowed to a trickle. When I went on the new diet, the drainage stopped. It was a little thing, to be sure, but I must tell you, it was joy to breathe through my unstopped nose 24 hours a day every day. I admit I found myself breathing through my mouth from sheer habit, but I worked on it. After all, who wants to look stupid?

Headaches. In my pre-allergy diet days, headaches occurred no more than three or four times a year. However, some of the headaches lasted for five or six days at a stretch. Over-the-counter pain relievers in double doses barely made it tolerable, but that is past now. Since the new diet I have had no headaches. The food(s) that caused the headaches remain a mystery.

Borderline anemia. (Chronic fatigue) At age 33, I complained to my doctor about chronic fatigue. I went to bed exhausted and slept soundly, but got up the next morning still tired.

I took a series of tests for diabetes, hypoglycemia and iron deficiency. All of this showed up normal results except for the iron text. I had borderline anemia. So the doctor prescribed iron pills as a dietary supplement and I followed his instructions until he retested me sometime later. The second test did not show one iota of improvement.

My fatigue became so bad, I could not project my voice at conferences and briefings. At annual physicals through the years, my blood tests continued to show the borderline anemia. Continued use of iron pills failed to help.

The brain is more powerful than most of us realize. The saying, "You are or become what you think about most" is true. I spent a good deal of time *thinking tired.*

I turned my life around in the tired department at about age 56; (33 to 56—it looks like I am a slow learner). This new approach of not thinking tired helped, but the afternoon energy fade still occurred. My blood test continued to show borderline anemia. That is the background before going into my new nutritional regimen. Now I feel like a new person, full of energy. In my work, I travel a lot, and as a result often come up short on sleep. Despite this, I continue to function at a high level without having a midafternoon energy fade.

Weight control. At age nineteen, I attained my full height of 5 feet 11 inches, and weighed 165 pounds; 175 at age thirty.

As the years went by, my weight crept up. At age 38, I topped out at 198 pounds.

I managed to get down to 190 before becoming a heart patient, then I lost thirty more pounds. Later, my weight crept back up from 160 to 172. To my great pleasure, with the food allergy diet, my weight dropped back to 165 within one week, without counting calories. As of this writing, eighteen months later, my weight is still rock solid at 165. It does not seem to matter how much or how little I eat, I still maintain my weight. This seems to stem from avoiding the foods I am allergic to and not being constipated. To me not worrying about weight control is nice.

Cold hands and feet. From age 35, this nuisance continued until the change in my diet.

Prostatic enlargement. This difficulty first appeared at about age 36, diagnosed during an Air Force annual physical. The doctor said my prostate was hardened and inflamed, and prescribed some antibiotics. When I asked "what happens if the medication does not work?" the doctor answered "I guess you'll learn to live with it." And that is exactly what I did—live with it.

At about age 45, drinking alcoholic beverages resulted in a sharp pain within two minutes as though somebody used an ice pick on my prostate. I quit drinking altogether for about three years.

My annual physicals continued to show a hardened and inflamed prostate. The condition advanced to the point it seriously interfered with passing water.

At about age 55, a urologist gave me an examination, and guess what? I had a hardened and inflamed prostate gland.

The doctor prescribed more antibiotics, and said if the medication did not work, I would need an operation. One week later I went for a checkup and discovered the antibiotics had not worked. The following week, my secretary told me her father suffered with the same problem. He took a regimen of one zinc tablet three times a day for 30 days and the problem cleared up. Since I did not relish the prospect of going under the knife, I thought it worth a try. Miracle of miracles, it worked. The subsequent examination revealed my prostate to be soft, and not inflamed. This was my early introduction to the success of a nutritional supplement, but I failed to grasp the full meaning of the situation; like maybe, some of my *other* health concerns might be diet related.

Diverticulitis, first diagnosed at age 38. The doctor told me it was unusual for that early age. My doctor, a young Air Force flight surgeon, gave me a proctoscope examination.

For the uninitiated, the proctoscope is an instrument for examining the colon. It is a round metal tube about three-quarter inches in diameter and approximately 14 inches long which is inserted in the anus to inspect the condition of the colon. In recent years medical science developed a flexible tube approximately 44 inches long employing fibre optics technology. The longer instrument facilitates the visual inspection of the full length of the colon which helps the doctor to prescribe the correct therapy or drug. The examination confirmed the diverticulitis. The doctor told me to eat nothing but bland, cooked foods; no raw fruit or vegetables.

Later in life with another diverticulitis episode and another doctor, I learned milk is a primary irritant to the lower digestive track and colon for many people, including me.

Yet another diverticulitis attack occurred about twenty years after my first episode, that preceded this new awareness of good nutrition. Because of my now superior knowledge of what caused it, rather than bother the doctor, I simply stopped drinking milk. As expected, in about two weeks, everything got back to normal. But this time I decided to stay off milk altogether. After one month of abstinence, my continual sinus drainage slowed down to a trickle. Also, the soreness in my finger joints lessened to a noticeable degree. It got me to *thinking* of the impact a change in my diet made.

Nocturnal leg and foot cramps. The cramps started about age 40 and got progressively worse, to a point of it becoming a nightly occurrence. Sometimes I suffered two or three painful episodes per night. The change of diet completely eliminated this nuisance within 60 days. I believe the vitamin and mineral supplements made the difference. I kept hearing the story—"once you have nocturnal leg and foot cramps, you will have them for life." I do not believe it anymore!

Cold sores. This nuisance started about age forty. I did not go to the doctor until the sores started getting into my nasal passages (about age 52). The doctor specified a prescription ointment, but the darn stuff did not do much good.

Two things happened to change this situation. First, I learned the application of an ice cube to the sore accelerated the healing process (like putting an ice cube on the sore). This particular gem of knowledge predates the food allergy testing and resultant diet by four or five years. The cold sores started to occur less and less as a result of my new diet. I only had the sores at about two month intervals. Four months into my new diet, the sores disappeared altogether. I suspect the vitamin and/or mineral supplementation to be the reason for improvement.

Muscle spasms. My first severe muscle spasm in the middle of my back resembled a heart attack, supposedly a result of stress. I believe the lack of vitamins or minerals may have played a part in the spasms. The doctor said I had a muscle spasm and not a heart attack and sent me home for bed rest. That turned out to be about 24 hours of straight sleeping (no getting up for the bathroom). Subsequently, I never had another spasm so severe, although from time to time I did have recurring muscle spasms of lesser intensity; but now they have disappeared altogether.

Dry nasal passages. This condition is an aggravation. As I recall, it started about age forty. I tried to alleviate the dryness by splashing tap water up my nose. I thought I had ruined something in my system as a result of heavy smoking in earlier years.

About 45 days into the new food allergy diet regimen, I noticed my nasal passages were no longer dry. They remained moist 24 hours a day.

Dry eyes. This means the normal tearing action is not there to keep the eyeballs lubricated. When the doctor asked if I had any dry eye problem, I answered, "no." To make sure, the doctor made an appointment with an opthamologist whose tests proved I *did* have dry eyes.

Why did I answer *no* when the doctor asked about my eyes? At about age 41, I started using eye drops on a daily basis. Within a year, rather than having a soothing effect, the drops irritated my eyes. So, I substituted tap water. I attributed the dry eye condition to improper use of the eye drops (these eye drops were not artificial tears).

The week following the examination, my dry eye condition became severe. The artificial tears soothed, but the desired effect usually lasted less than 30 minutes.

Again, the change in my diet, which included vitamin and mineral supplements, resulted in the return of my natural tears within 60 days. Another clear-cut case of success.

Hemorrhoids. Hemorrhoids showed up on the scene in my early forties as a direct result of being constipated and straining to have a bowel movement. I suspect this same scenario is the prime contributor for the development of the diverticulitis mentioned earlier. I started taking artificial bulk to soften the stool and help with the bowel movement but I still had to strain. As a result of not being constipated anymore, the hemorrhoids disappeared; relief from another *aging* dysfunction.

Stomach ulcers. This is a good news/bad news story told with 20–20 hindsight. The ulcers happened in my second year of civilian life after leaving the military service. During the Christmas season, the secretaries brought in all sorts of goodies for a full week before the holiday vacation. I decided to relax, to forget weight control, and enjoy myself. Known as the "cookie bear," I could not eat just one cookie, but maybe one dozen would do. I especially favored brownies and fudge. So Christmas vacation came and I continued eating sweets, contrary to my pre-Christmas season eating habits. The second week in the new year, my stomach rebelled.

A trip to the doctor revealed I had the perfect symptoms of a stomach ulcer. At this time in my life, I habitually drank at least ten to twelve cups of coffee every day. The treatment prescribed:

- eat only bland, well-cooked foods
- drink whole milk (this predates my knowledge about the milk influence on diverticulitis)
- eliminate coffee and spices

After about six weeks of this regimen I returned to the doctor for a checkup. He said I looked good, and it was all right to go back to my regular diet but cut down to one or two cups of coffee per day. With the next cup of coffee, the first swallow felt like sulphuric acid. Who needs this pain I thought. I drank my last cup of coffee, more than 24 years ago—and my stomach still says "thank you." No more ulcers or minor stomach distress.

But alas, this is not the end of this episode. Yes, my stomach did clear up, but then severe pains showed up in my lower groin, a second bout with diverticulitis. The doctor recommended the same bland ulcer diet with milk. After a job relocation, I found a new doctor to treat my diverticulitis. The doctor's diet prescription—"stop drinking milk, but eat anything else that does not upset your stomach." I rapidly got better. The diverticulitis and associated pain completely disappeared in about ten days.

Later, I learned of my allergy to chocolate. Perhaps my Christmas holiday binge of chocolate goodies caused the ulcers.

The bad news is:

- Stomach ulcers and diverticulitis are no fun at all!

Now the good news:

- Apparently, my dietary indiscretion caused my ulcer problem, and I now know it is within my power to control.
- Milk is a primary cause of my diverticulitis. Now, milk is not on my diet, and consequently I have no more threat of developing diverticulitis.

Brittle nails. Obviously this condition is not life threatening, but it is an indication of something wrong. Many people told me this is a sure sign of a calcium deficiency. My brittle nail condition was greatly alleviated with the calcium supplementation to my diet.

Bursitis. I developed this affliction at age 56. I used a power sander to get rid of chipped and peeling paint on the outside of the house. I worked with the heavy sander over my head, which seemed to aggravate the shoulder condition. My doctor diagnosed the sore shoulder as bursitis, and gave me a shot of cortisone which worked wonders. The pain instantly subsided, and remained pain free for just one week. Then, when I was up and about it presented no pain. However, within thirty minutes after I went to bed, the pain became excruciating.

It took six months for the pain to decrease to tolerable levels. As I flexed my right shoulder, I could hear a popping sound and feel some pain. The change in my diet eliminated the popping and little pain remains when I flex my shoulder in a rotary motion. The restricted action in my right shoulder completely disappeared after two years of the food allergy diet regimen.

Arthritis in the finger joints. The soreness in my finger joints became noticeable in my mid-fifties. The soreness grew progressively worse. I thought this could be hereditary since my mother was severely crippled with arthritis in her hands. In my case, just before my food allergy discovery, at random times with the slightest movement two finger joints would make a loud popping noise. Pain would shoot up my arm as if under Chinese torture of some kind. Whether they popped or not, most of the finger joints felt sore and a knob began to develop on my left index finger which concerned me.

As I said earlier, this condition greatly improved when I gave up milk. Within 30 days of starting the food allergy diet, the popping and soreness almost disappeared; beef seemed to be the offending food. In another three months, my hands felt nearly normal; a little stiff, but without pain. Another victory over the *normal aging process*.

Dry mouth. This difficulty started my journey toward a new, nutritional life; *eating to live* instead of *living to eat*. In May, at age 60, this dry mouth condition coincided with another diverticulitis episode; getting both ends of the stick, painful in different ways.

The dry mouth condition returned periodically over the next week. Two weeks after the Carlisle trip, I decided to visit my family doctor. I thought he could fix anything, but I felt dumb telling him I had a dry mouth problem. I thought his response would be to take a drink of water. Later I learned he had three other cases in the past week.

My doctor called the dry mouth by the clinical name, *xerostomia*. The doctor said there is no known cure for xerostomia and all he could do is treat the symptoms. Specifically, this meant using an artificial saliva mouth spray—awful tasting stuff, although it is advertised to be tasteless. Sometimes it worked for one minute, the next time a half hour, or half of a day.

Additionally, my doctor advised me that xerostomia frequently is the precursor of collagen vascular disease, an inflammatory disorder involving joints, muscles, arteries and multiple organs, putting a good scare into me. My blood tests did not reveal any evidence of diabetes, or any other condition that might cause me to have a dry mouth. My doctor suspected some primary disorder of the salivary glands.

My friend Meg insisted I see Dr. J, a practicing chiropractor and nutritionist. Eventually, I did see him which led to the food allergy test and a change of diet and vitamin and mineral supplementation. My dry mouth condition substantially improved within 30 days, and returned to near normal within 90 days.

Continual belching and passing of foul smelling gas. I became a veritable volcano. I burbled and burped most of the time; and the awful smell! In the three to four years predating the change to the new diet, it became progressively worse. I became so concerned I asked my doctor about this condition but he did not give me any clue as to the cause.

You must have guessed the answer already. The new diet resolved this situation.

Hardening of the arteries (atherosclerosis). Diagnosed at age 55 during my annual physical. A resting EKG test did not reveal the problem but the treadmill stress test did. As a result, the doctor prescribed a drug. It slowed down my heart beat, and lowered my energy level.

I changed my diet by eating less fat and meat. Additionally, I started exercising on a regular basis. I walked two miles, twice a day and lost 25 pounds in three months. However my angina attacks came with increasing frequency and severity. It seemed as though I lived on nitroglycerin pills.

Finally, my doctor decided to do an angiogram. As preparation for the test, I again underwent a stress test, which revealed the same heart deficiency. I got the angiogram done with a catheter injected into the main artery in the groin area. They pumped dye along the way as they pushed the catheter toward the heart which allowed them to see the condition of the artery and how the heart valves functioned. These things turned out to be normal. Consequently, my doctor took me off medication and declared I did not need bypass surgery.

I did not realize how much the medication dragged me down by slowing my pulse rate. After going off the drugs, it felt as though I had one large shot of adrenaline, lasting for a month.

Maybe a miracle happened to reverse my heart condition but I personally subscribe to the theory that I did not suffer from severe angina episodes until after I took drugs to slow down my heart. I believe I may have been run down when treated as a heart patient. I was fortunate not to have any blockages, nothing more than hardening of the arteries.

Cosmetic appearance. When I did not look good, I did not feel good. Five things changed for the better: the color of my teeth; the color and texture of my skin; the sparkle of my eyes; the dandruff disappeared; and my hair now looks alive.

Before the new diet, the color of my teeth resembled old piano keys, ivory yellow. Some people thought I was a heavy smoker because of the color, but I quit more than 25 years earlier. About 30 days into my new diet I noticed the color of the tips of my teeth changed to white. As time passed the white kept creeping toward the gum line.

The color of my skin once had the gray pallor of an elderly person. Also, my face had an unhealthy oily feel; not part dry and part oily, but just plain oily. With the change in diet, my skin soon looked and felt healthy with a pinkish color like Li'l Abner's hammus alabamus.

My eyes always seemed to appear dull—at least that is what many of my friends told me. Of course I knew that without their help by looking in the mirror. The change in diet brought a sparkle back to my eyes.

Dandruff continued to be a problem most of my adult life. After about one year into the new diet, the dandruff nearly disappeared, and after two years, totally gone.

On several occasions old friends exclaimed, with apparent sincerity, "You are growing younger—how do you do it?" The Bible says: "all is vanity—all is vanity." It may be vanity, but I must tell you—it is *serendipity* to me.

After the first eighteen months on the new diet, I believed I mastered the problem of slowing down the aging process. I experienced more than my fair share of success. However, this euphoria did not last. There were some reversals and more lessons to be learned. Diet, including vitamin and mineral supplements and exercise, are only a part of the answer. Some other items needing attention include dental hygiene, proper spinal alignment, recognition of digestive system dysfunction, and the effects of the environment.

CHAPTER 4

Health Profile Analysis

Chapter 3 talked about my physical profile and the miraculous transformation. This chapter presents the same chronological order, with a description of my activities and diet so my background/environment might be examined to determine its influence on my health. This is addressed in ten-year segments so I may analyze the cumulative effect, a revelation even to myself!

My conditions and ailments totaled 23. Out of the 23, I do not expect to have trouble with more than two to four because I now *eat to live.* I will discuss this further at the end of this chapter.

Most of my problems are cumulative up to age 60. I had the usual assortment of childhood diseases including measles, mumps and scarlet fever, but these are not included in my analysis.

I came from a family of five boys born in Glenn Ellyn, Ill. My father died of cancer of the pancreas when I was six. My little brother David and I went to live with our maternal grandparents in Topeka, Kansas. Two years later, my mother and the other brothers joined us. Shortly after mother's arrival, we left the grandparents to live in our own rented house. The depression days were tough times for everybody. My mother taught school at Roosevelt Junior High, and received a monthly starting salary of $96, later increased to $106.

The first decade in this story starts with the age bracket of ten to twenty years. I can recall chronic constipation and getting up once or twice at night to urinate.

We lived on a small thirteen-acre farm just outside town. Our diet consisted mostly of fresh fruits, vegetables, fresh milk, and chicken. However, mother served meat only four or five meals a week.

My activities for the ten-to-twenty decade included the completion of junior and senior high school. I was not a particularly good student, as I thought school to be boring. I played hooky for a spell and wound up with a C-plus average. After school I worked on the farm, milked the cows, fed the chickens and helped with the garden. I had a paper route from age 12 to 17. Most of the time, I delivered the morning paper. This meant getting up about 4 a.m. to keep my 180 to 200 customers happy. The paper route delivery was always on foot. For recreation in the spring, summer and fall, I went on long hikes or bicycle rides. I spent five summers with two different uncles on their farms. Activities there included driving the tractor, operating a combine, and the usual chores of feeding the animals and milking the six to fourteen cows. I remember I seemed to be a perpetual motion machine full of energy.

One time, my brother David and I started at noon on Saturday to see how far we could hike. We used the Boy Scout method of jogging 50 paces, then walking 50 paces. We covered about 45 miles between noon and midnight. We came home to a very worried mother, and couldn't understand her anger even though we had not told her we were going for a hike.

Now on to the next decade. As you recall, I started out with constipation and urination problems. Now add one more—sinus drainage; this was no big deal except for some related bronchitis that I will talk about later.

I am fudging a bit here on the twenty–thirty decade, because I joined the Army at eighteen, and that part is included here for convenience of telling the story.

I joined the Army with my older brother Paul. My diet changed radically. The Army menu had meat three times a day, and dessert for lunch and dinner. The Army served fruit and vegetables, mostly canned, except for potatoes; I know the potatoes were fresh because I peeled enough of them on KP.

At age nineteen, I attended enlisted pilots' flying school. At the graduation banquet celebration, a friend and I tried to drink all the liquor in Texas. I overindulged to an extreme, vomiting blood before completing the evening celebration. It makes me curious whether this episode had damaging effects on one or more of my body parts, particularly the liver and kidneys.

Before the end of my nineteenth year, I began my overseas tour in India as a U.S. Army Air Corps pilot flying C-47 aircraft over "the Hump" between India and China. The diet again changed radically to British rations—beef (Indian water buffalo) for lunch and dinner seven days a week, no milk, and rancid, canned butter. I started to drink coffee made from pure chicory. I came back to the United States at age twenty-one to a steady diet of meat three times a day. I also picked up the habit of eating junk food and drinking beer and hard liquor (not to excess, except occasionally on party night). I started smoking at nineteen.

I enjoyed excellent health during this period except for a severe case of bronchitis, apparently developed from the sinus drainage. My doctor told me to lie over the edge of the bed with my head almost touching the floor fifteen minutes out of every hour during my waking hours. On the third day of this exercise, I coughed up a round mass of hardened mucous about the size of a golf ball.

I also developed pneumonia at the close of my overseas tour and came back home on medical rotation. I fully recovered after two weeks in the Miami regional hospital.

After the return to duty, I ferried just about every type aircraft in the inventory. The deliveries took me all over the United States as well as Europe, Africa, Australia, South America, and many of the islands in the Southwest Pacific.

I married at age twenty-two and soon had two handsome sons. My wife was a good companion, lover, mother, accomplished homemaker and cook, so I lived the good life.

Now we move into the thirty–forty decade. At the start of this time period, the cumulative score consisted of three health issues: urinary disorder, constipation, and sinus drainage, none of which were of any real significance. The thirty–forty period added seven more.

I started to suffer infrequent severe headaches. My wife complained of my cold hands and feet.

Other new health concerns included enlarged, inflamed prostate, diverticulitis, nocturnal leg cramps and chronic fatigue. The chronic fatigue persisted from about age thirty-three to fifty-six. The fatigue disappeared when I stopped *thinking tired*.

My weight crept up to 198; this from 165 at age twenty; and 175 at age thirty. My dietary habits of eating three meals a day with meat, and having desserts five out of seven evening meals continued. I attacked my weight problem with several fad diets, but none of them brought success. It seemed my weight would end up two or three pounds heavier with every diet change.

During this period, I quit smoking as a matter of survival. Either quit, or meet an early grave, I thought, as I smoked two to three packs a day. My early morning cigarette cough cleared up after a couple of months. I also took up jogging for two years. I jogged about one mile, seven days a week, early in the morning. This did not seem to have any positive effect on my health.

Entering into the forty–fifty period with the scoreboard at eleven, my problems increased by six—cold sores, muscle spasms, dry nasal passages, dry eyes, hemorrhoids and stomach ulcer.

By the early forties, I had transitioned from the military service into civilian life and picked up some bad habits. I became a daily drinker, slowly but steadily increasing the intake. Starting with a one-shot bourbon drink, it soon became two. Then the double shots replaced the two single-shot drinks, and then three double shot drinks. I finally quit. In about one week, it seemed as though a fog began to lift from my brain, a most remarkable sensation and a welcomed feeling.

My stomach ulcer that occurred at age forty motivated me to give up coffee. And of course I learned the lesson of moderation when it comes to sweets. I know I will have only myself to blame should I develop another ulcer.

In the fifty–sixty time period, things really added up. A cumulative score of sixteen to age fifty with seven more to come in the ensuing decade. Five additional items included brittle nails, flatulence, bursitis, arthritis and dry mouth. Another item to be included in this list was hardening of the arteries. The degrading cosmetic appearance was additive over the years and included in this decade for accounting purposes.

By now, you must consider me decrepit. Quite to the contrary, most of these things I took in stride as the *normal aging process*. However, the continued chronic fatigue did nothing to improve my outlook on life.

My eating habits during the early part of this decade underwent a slow evolutionary change. First, I gave up meat for breakfast, except for Sunday morning. Later, I gave up meat for lunch. Also, I cut down on the meat portion from six to eight ounces per serving, to four ounces. During this same period, I cut back from having desserts several times a week, to two or three times. *The Pritikin Program for Diet and Exercise* had a significant influence upon me. I will discuss the radical change in diet in detail later in the book.

My physical habits during this period changed as well. As a heart patient, I learned the value of regular exercise and its contribution to staying fit and healthy. I now walk about four miles and do about fifteen minutes of calisthenics six or seven days a week. Additionally, I work in a high-rise office building and I walk up the nine flights of stairs two at a time.

As a result of changing my lifestyle, I feel as physically fit as I did in earlier years.

The collection of my health concerns included changes in cosmetic appearance that I discussed earlier, but that is vanity. Now the recapitulation:

age span	number of new problems	cumulation
10–20	2	2
20–30	1	3
30–40	7	10
40–50	6	16
50–60	7	23

My scoreboard says twenty-three, but nineteen of those items are not expected to recur. The score of continued concerns is four:

1. I still get up once or twice a night to go to the bathroom
2. I still have diverticulosis and am subject to diverticulitis, but being rid of constipation and not drinking milk lessens the probability
3. I have a trace of bursitis but it is diminishing
4. the dry mouth is much improved, but still not fully recovered.

Gone are the chronic fatigue, headaches, arthritic pain, dry nose and eyes, stomach ulcers, hemorrhoids, weight control difficulties, and constipation.

CHAPTER 5

Food Allergy Testing

Before testing, I did not have the remotest understanding of food allergies.

The first test revealed a total of nineteen items. The regimen specified the allergy diet for ninety days to reset my digestive system to zero, specifically, to eliminate the lingering adverse effects from the food to which I showed some intolerance. After ninety days, the doctor told me to start taking one food at a time to assess the reaction.

When I tried beef the first time after a ninety day fast from all red meat, the reactions were immediate—

- my arthritic pain in my hands reappeared within ten minutes.
- I became constipated, suffered three days before the next bowel movement.
- I had trouble with flatulence and foul-smelling gas, symptomatic of putrefaction rather than digestion.

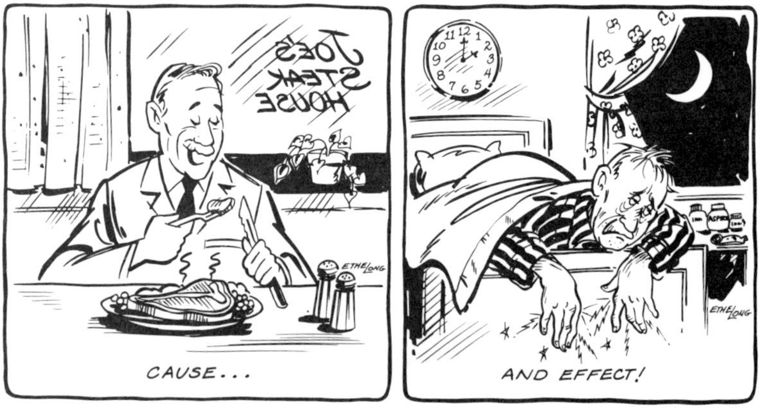

CAUSE . . . AND EFFECT!

Over a span of time, I had different types of food allergy tests done. Additionally, I had a skin test to detect sensitivity to a few chemicals. I will treat these individually, outlining the procedures I went through, and a word or two about the results achieved:

- cytotoxic food allergy test
- CIRA—Cellular Immune Response Assay
- intradermal food allergy test
- pulse testing for food allergies
- intradermal testing for chemical allergies
- observation of food allergy test results
- examples of severe limitations that some food allergies can impose

CYTOTOXIC FOOD ALLERGY TESTING

My friend Meg referred me to Dr. J, a Chiropractor/ Nutritionist. It took a couple of weeks of debating with myself before I finally made up my mind to visit him. In my initial appointment, I put the question to him rather bluntly, "What qualifies you to be a nutritionist?" He went on to explain a number of nutrition courses are a basic requirement in the formal education for chiropractors. Further, he said that good nutrition is considered to be one of the important elements in chiropractic treatment. More about this in Chapter 8.

Dr. J said he had particularly good luck in combining food allergy testing/diet with vitamin and mineral supplements. My family doctor told me *there is no known cure* for dry eyes. This miserable condition served as the spark to search for the cure. Did a food allergy contribute to my dry mouth and dry eyes? It was this condition that brought me to this position of searching for the answer.

I already learned from Dr. Henry Beiler in *Food is Your Best Medicine* that the body is a chemical factory. I must have done something wrong to mess it up. If any recovery were possible it would have to be from *getting right* with my chemical factory. Elimination of the foods I could not tolerate seemed the smart thing to do. At this time, I had no idea of my allergies. As far as I was concerned, I could consume anything but milk, but the food allergy tests revealed something quite different.

I decided to proceed with Dr. J's recommended approach, the steps to my initial success were:

First:	The cytotoxic food allergy test
Second:	Preparation for taking diet supplements by using pyrodoxine to purge the toxins stored in my system (predominantly the colon as I understand it). This procedure involves taking several pyrodoxine tablets over a short period of time.
Third:	Eliminate the food allergy items from my diet
Fourth:	Add minerals and vitamin supplements.

In about thirty days on the food allergy diet, the acute nature of my dry eyes and dry mouth subsided. In ninety days both my eyes and mouth seemed nearly normal. Some unexpected serendipity came along with this:—

- my dry nose cleared up! Here I thought the dry nose to be the direct result of the tobacco habit in earlier years, aging, or a combination of the two.
- Beef was identified as the culprit to my arthritic pain, chronic constipation, flatulence and putrefaction problems.

The information Dr. J gave me indicated the cytotoxic test is the best known method to determine food and chemical intolerance. The cytotoxic test is a laboratory procedure first described by Arthur Black, M.D. at the Washington University School of Medicine in St. Louis.

The laboratory procedure consists of observing the reactions of the living white blood cells, red blood cells and platelets after the blood is exposed to foods, dyes and other chemicals. If the cells remain uniformly round, indicating a healthy state, that food is not harmful. However, if the shape of the cells change, become paralyzed or disintegrate, that indicates a food intolerance or food allergy.

There are documented cases indicating diet and allergies are a prime factor in "learning disabilities." Some children are physically sound and bright but act disturbed and hyperactive from food allergies. Children with a food intolerance often show the symptoms of faulty memory, poor concentration and even poor visual and perceptual skills.

Other physical distress caused by food allergies can include:

- chronic fatigue
- sinus problems
- obesity and food addiction
- hyperactivity
- arthritis
- high blood pressure
- frequent colds
- depression
- confusion and memory loss
- mental problems
- mood swings
- stomach and bowel problems
- insomnia
- cold hands and feet

The cytotoxic food test has the advantage that a maximum number of foods can be tested from one blood sample from the patient.

The preparation is to have nothing to eat or drink for twelve hours before the test. A blood sample is taken and shipped off to the lab for analysis and testing of 134 items. The technical jargon below describing this test is taken from information provided by the Bio Medical Science Laboratory, Los Angeles, California.

"The cytotoxic test, leukocyte sensitivity index, is a laboratory procedure which consists of observing the reaction of the patient's living white blood cells to pure antigen extract dilutions. The procedure consists of centrifugation for a minimum of 45 minutes at slow speed, exposure of white blood cells to antigens that have been fixed to microscopic slides, then incubation. They are then examined by a trained technician for disintefraction and vacoulization of the segmented neutrophils. The panel of tests includes one hundred thirty-four antigens with patient controls

The grading categories of the test are:

N-negative, S-suspect, P-positive

The list of my allergies from this test are noted:

	S	*P*
raisin grape	X	
cane sugar	X	
wheat		X
cashew nut	X	
baker's yeast		X
brewer's yeast		X
kidney bean		X
peanut		X
coffee		X
tomato		X
green peppers	X	
sesame		X
cocoa, chocolate		X
brazil nut	X	
beef	X	
pork		X
evaporated milk		X
yogurt	X	
*(cow's milk not tested)		

In the food allergy elimination diet the "S", "suspect" items are treated the same as "P", "positive." In other words, you do not get to eat those foods.

Dr. J gave me bibliography on the subject of cytotoxic tests. Investigation at the local Veteran's Hospital library prompted the following letter to the cytotoxic testing laboratory.

Dear Dr. C:

On 20 July, you ran a cytotoxic test for me. My question is, how accurate is this procedure? Dr. J tells me it is near to one hundred percent accurate. However, articles I read from a bibliography did not agree with his position. Enclosed is a copy of a controlled test. In part it says, "The cytotoxic food test was not found to be an accurate method for diagnosing atopic reactions to food. Claims that the test correlate with other untoward reactions to foods (e.g. headaches, diarrhea, fatigue) could not be corroborated. The test itself is time consuming, dependent on subjective interpretations, and inconsistency results when repetitive runs are performed on the same patient."

I want to believe the cytotoxic test is valid and accurate. Please provide me with information giving clinical proof that this testing procedure is mature and worth using as a diagnostic tool.

Yours truly,
Frank K. Mattson

The response is summarized by the following points:

- The methodology and protocol developed by Arthur Black, M.D. was refined by W. Bryant, M.D. at Washington University School of Medicine. It is the only accurate and acceptable methodology.
- Superficial examination of your enclosure, several variables are noted: (1) the antigen dilution of 1:4 is too concentrated; (2) amount of antigen to buffy coat is unclear; (3) amount of serum and water mixture is improper.
- This article also states the test was inaccurate for atopic individuals. This test was never intended to diagnose IgE mediated conditions, rather those of individual maladaptive reactions.

I made an attempt to claim the Cytotoxic Food Allergy Test on my group health insurance. This is the rejection notice.

Dear Mr. Mattson:

We have received this claim. We regret that we are unable to make payment at this time for reasons indicated below. Please refer to the section of your booklet/certificate entitled "expenses not covered" or "General Limitations": "Not necessary care and treatment of an illness, injury or pregnancy". If you feel your claim should have been covered, you may ask to have it reviewed within 60 days of receipt of this letter. Please state the reasons, etc.

We will notify you of the final decision within 60 days of receipt of your request.

I did choose to make a reclama:

Dear Sir:

This letter is in response to your letter of September 15. My statement of reclama is presented below.

On May 20 I was advised by my family physician that I had contracted a condition known as dry mouth and dry eyes. He prescribed artificial saliva and artificial tears which did nothing but relieve the symptoms. The condition persisted and gradually worsened.

As I reflected on the problem, I came to believe it was nutrition related. Consequently, I decided to have a cytotoxic food test done after some investigation. After learning the results of the cytotoxic allergy test, I have avoided the foods indicated. In a short time my condition improved. I do not have to use the artificial help except on infrequent occasions. I offer this as evidence that avoiding the foods the cytotoxic food test revealed is having results. Whether the total condition of the xerostomia will be relieved will only be known in a matter of time.

I consulted further with the doctor on October 12. He advised me the dry mouth is frequently a precursor associated with collagen vascular disease, an inflamatory disorder involving muscles, joints, arteries, and multiple organs. He said it was too early to tell whether the soreness in my finger joints is a sufficient sign to indicate the disease is beginning to stir. The soreness in all of my other finger knuckle joints has subsided since mid-August. I submit this as another sign of the validity of the cytotoxic test.

My conviction after having talked to my doctor is that it would be only a matter of time before the collagen vascular disease sets in unless I take some action to ward it off. The early signs show success. Consequently, it appears I will avoid an early deterioration in my health; and the necessity of making significant claims against my group health insurance. In view of the above, your re-evaluation of my claim would be appreciated.

Yours very truly,
Frank K Mattson

(*collagen vascular disease is an insoluble protein fiber that forms in the joints and veins.) My reclama did not meet with success.

CIRA-CELLULAR IMMUNE RESPONSE ASSAY

Patient preparation—overnight fasting is required, but medication need not be suspended.

Preparation of the blood sample—must be received by the laboratory within twenty-four hours. Refrigeration of the sample is not required, but temperature extremes should be avoided.

A comprehensive panel of ninety-seven foods tested with the CIRA technique and the CIRA scores correspond to the increasing extent of morphological changes due to the formations of allergen/IgG antibody complexes on the neutrophil surface.

Score	0;	Negative, 1–4% morphological change
Score	1+;	Suspicious, 5–10% morphological change
Score	2+;	Positive, 11–20% morphological change
Score	3+;	Positive, 21–40% morphological change
Score	4+;	Positive, 41–60% morphological change
Score	5+;	Positive, 61–80% morphological change

This test cost $195 in 1984 and was paid by my group health insurance company without any questions.

The CIRA tests and intradermal food allergy test did have a close correlation. This will be shown later.

INTRADERMAL ALLERGY TEST

I backslid on taking my vitamin supplements starting in February 1986 with bad results in July 1986. My dry mouth and dry eyes returned. By this time, Dr. J added a registered dietitian to his staff who advised me that the most probable cause is a lack of Vitamin A and the multi-B vitamin complex. Next I proceeded with the intradermal testing to determine the validity of the cytotoxic and CIRA analysis.

In the intradermal test, the prerequisite is to keep a food diary. After two weeks, this is summarized as indicated in Figures 5–1A and 1B. This then becomes the basis for the first battery of tests; the tests for food allergies are limited to fifty. Additional testing costs more money.

INTRADERMAL FOOD TESTING

MARK NUMBER OF TIMES INGESTED
FOR A TWO-WEEK PERIOD

Totals

EXAMPLE: 10 - turkey - ~~1111~~ ~~1111~~

Totals

MEATS:
Chicken 11
Ham 1
Eggs 111
Lamb 1

FISH:
Mackeral 11
Tuna 111
Halibut 1
Grouper 1

SHELLFISH:
Clams 11
Shrimp 1
Scallop 111
Oyster 1
Lobster 11

Totals

FRUITS:
Apple ~~1111~~ ~~1111~~
Cranberry 1
Cherries ~~1111~~
Grapes ~~1111~~ ~~1111~~ 11
Grapefruit 111
Orange ~~1111~~ 1
Plum 111
Pear 111
Peach ~~1111~~
Pineapple 111
Strawberry 1
Banana ~~1111~~ 111

NUTS:
Almond ~~1111~~ ~~1111~~ 1
Pecan ~~1111~~ ~~1111~~ 1
Walnut 11
Peanuts ~~1111~~ ~~1111~~

FIGURE 5-1A

Examination of Figure 5-1A will show I went overboard with fruit, so I ingested too much fructose—in other words, sugar. My energy level was going down the drain, but I did not know why. When my dietician saw this, she knew why. I cut back on the fruit, and my energy level increased. This I liked. I now limit myself to one fruit per day or one glass of fruit juice.

VEGETABLES:
Broccoli 11
Lettuce 𝍸
Beets 1
Carrot 111
Celery 𝍸
Cucumber 𝍸

LEGUMES:
Mustard 111
Black Eyed Peas 11
Green Peas 11
Navy Beans 11
Stringbean 111
Onion 11
Irish Potato 𝍸 𝍸 111
Tomato 1

SWEETNERS:
Cane Sugar 11

OILS:
None

CHEESE:
Cheddar 1
Cottage 111

DRINK:
Beer
Wine

ADDITIVES:
None

SEASONING:
None

OTHER:
Amaranth 1
Cantelope 11
Margarine 𝍸 𝍸 11
Ice Cream 1

GRAINS:
Barley 1
Oats 𝍸
Rice 𝍸 111
Wheat 𝍸 𝍸 𝍸 𝍸 1
Yeast—Bakers 𝍸 𝍸 111
Yeast—Brewers 1

FIGURE 5-1B

As with most medical laboratory testing, there is a certain routine that must be followed. My instructions stated:

- Do not take any medications at least two (2) days prior to your testing except medications specifically approved by this office. If there are any medications in question that you feel are important that you must take, please seek advice from this clinic.
- The Screening Intradermal Pin Prick Test takes approximately two hours. The Screening Intradermal Food Test

and any special Intradermal Tests take approximately one hour each.

- If your test is in the morning, before lunch, please have a light breakfast. If your test is after lunch, in the afternoon, you may have a full breakfast but a light lunch.
- Always wear a short sleeve shirt or blouse that fits loosely around your arms so that we may roll the sleeves over your shoulders.
- The cost of your tests will be $175.

While undergoing this battery of tests, I was in the same room as a young woman being tested for her sensitivity to tobacco. After the first pinprick test with tobacco allergen, she became incoherent and had difficulty breathing. Her situation appeared desperate. The doctor kept giving her different strengths of the antigen about every five minutes. On the sixth try she snapped out of it and regained a normal composure—although obviously emotionally drained.

The strength of the tobacco antigen that brought this woman back to reality became the prescription to desensitize her to tobacco. Apparently the smokers in her workplace caused her harm. This spectacular episode showed cause and treatment of an allergy.

My tests were dull and routine, however, the intradermal test revealed a close correlation to the CIRA test taken earlier as indicated below.

ITEM	1984 CIRA	1986 INTRADERMAL
Grapes	X	X
Chicken	X	X
Eggs	X	X
Cabbage	X	X
Carrots	X	X
Corn	X	X
Lettuce	X	X

Pinto Beans	X	X
Tomatoes	X	X
Soybeans	X	X
Pecans	X	not tested
String Beans	X	X
Safflower	X	not tested
Pork	X	X

In summary, 28 percent of tested items revealed an allergic reaction. That high percentage was compounded by eggs, corn, tomatoes, and soybeans identified as allergic. These items are used in many other foods. Consequently, if I observed the results of these findings, my diet would be severely limited. To illustrate the point, a listing of foods that eggs, soybeans, and corn are found in is depicted in Figures 5-2, 5-3, and 5-4 respectively.

FOODS CONTAINING EGG

Breads
Macaroons
Marshmallows
Sherbets
Pancake Flours
Waffle Mixes
Boiled Dressings
Salad Dressings
Cocoa Drinks (malted)
Meat Loaf
Sausages
Pastas
Soups:
  consommes
  noodle

Ice Cream
Icings (cakes & desserts)
Cakes
Puddings
Meringues
Pretzels
Batters for French Frying
Hollandaise Sauce
Egg Nog
Macaroni
Meat Jellies
Protein Drinks
Spaghetti

FIGURE 5-2

FOODS CONTAINING SOYBEANS

Soybean is used in many products. The main categories are flour, oil, milk, and nuts. Each year new products are released in the market containing soybean. Again, read the label—if you are allergic.

Breads
Cakes
Biscuits
Shortenings
Soyflour
Pastries

Butter Substitutes
Cereals
Dry Milk Substitutes
Pork Link Sausage

Lunch Meats
Soy Sprouts
Soy Nuts
Chinese Dishes

Soups
Chinese Foods
Soybean Noodles
Spaghetti

Ice Cream
Custards
Nut Candies

Protein Drinks
Coffee Substitutes
Milk Substitutes
Dry Lemonade Mix
Coffee Creamer

Oriental Sauces
Oil Dressings
Imitation Bacon Bits

Candles
Lecithin
Massage Creams
Glycerine
Lubricating Oil
Lamp Oil
Grease
Fish Food
Blankets & Cloth
Linoleum
Polishes
Varnish, paints & enamels
Printing Ink
Paper Sizing
Fertilizer
Nitroglycerine
Paper Finishes

FIGURE 5–3

FOODS CONTAINING CORN

Baking Mixes
Baking Powders
Bleached Wheat Flour
Cakes
Cookies
Powdered Sugar
Graham Crackers

Bacon
Batters for Frying
Corn Flakes
Frying Fats
Grits
Jams & Jellies

Cheeses
Sandwich Spreads
Fritos
Hams (tenderized or cured)
Meats (Bologna, Sausage)
Tortillas

Rice (coated)
Soups (vegetable & creamed)

Cream Pies
Ice Creams

Aspirins & Other Tablets
Chewing Gum
Cough Syrups
Gelatin Capsules
Similac
Soy Bean Milks
Vanilla
Vitamins—Tablets & Capsules
Suppositories

Glucose Products
Corn Syrup
Corn Sugar

Ketchups
Salad Dressings
Sauces for Meats
Sauces for Sundaes
French Dressings
Gravies

Ales & Beer
Carbonated Beverages
Bourbon Whiskies
Grape Juice (check label)

FIGURE 5–4

PULSE TESTING

Dr. Coca first discovered the correlation of the measured pulse rate with food allergies. Coca's book, *The Pulse Test,* outlines his experience and application of this technique. He came to recognize food allergies are a prime cause of sickness. The discovery of the pulse correlation for diagnoses would "revolutionize medicine." He made that statement about 35 years ago. Today it is hard to find anybody who understands and takes this seriously.

Coca's wife was suddenly stricken and in continual distress from angina pectoris, unable to function well for about three years. His approach to treating his wife had not met with success until by accident he discovered his wife's resting pulse rate seemed to be adversely affected by a certain food. This affectation was repeatable. Understanding this, he tested her reaction to other foods. Having noted the results, he suggested that she not eat any of the offending foods. *Her mysterious malady rapidly dissipated and she returned to normal functioning after adjusting her diet.*

There are different routines to using the RPR to determine your reaction to foods. The way I do it is to wait until my digestive system has processed all of the food I have eaten last. I allow at least eight hours. I usually do the test first thing in the morning. I keep a log and measure my RPR before eating the first food, then re-measure the RPR in fifteen minutes, and then thirty minutes. If there is no change, no allergy is indicated. If however, the RPR raised five to ten points this is a positive allergic reaction. If the RPR does not indicate a positive reaction, I proceed with additional foods until a positive reaction is noted. At that time, testing must be discontinued until the digestive system re-zeroed.

By the pulse testing method I set out to validate the CIRA and intradermal skin test. I have made the following observations:

- pecans and pinto beans—confirmed as allergic
- safflower oil, corn, grapes and carrots—not confirmed by the pulse test
- sweet potatoes—confirmed as allergic but did not show up in previous tests. This begs the question of "am I allergic to the sweet potato or the chemicals with which it is treated?" I cannot answer without further investigation.

INTRADERMAL CHEMICAL TEST

I completed the testing in August 1986 for four chemical reactions: BHT, BHA, petro chemicals, formaldehyde. BHT and BHA are preservatives commonly used in boxed foods such as cereals. I tested positive for all items except petro chemicals. The prescription directed one drop per day under the tongue to desensitize me to BHT and formaldehyde. When I asked how long I would have to do this, I got the answer, "the rest of your life."

My dry eye irritation (dry eyes) returned about the time I discovered my allergic reaction to formaldehyde. I had just completed wallpapering my entire house, including all closets and the garage. So you ask, where is formaldehyde used? It is used in vinyl wallpaper as well as the following:

- nail polish
- vinyl of any other sort, including automobile upholstery
- shampoo
- formica
- paper—grocery bags, wax paper, tissue, newsprint
- plywood
- insecticides and fungicides
- plastics of all description—toys, eyeglass frames and lenses, cooking utensils . . .
- detergents
- rugs, drapes, flame resistant clothes
- disinfectants, air fresheners

In our world, we are surrounded by formaldehyde. By keeping careful mental notes I determined that my eye irritation symptomatic of dry eyes, is in reality a reaction to the formaldehyde. When I am outside in the fresh air I have no problem. In the house or in the car where formaldehyde is present, the irritation returns. This action/reaction is repeatable.

Interestingly, the determination of the allergic reaction is done by observation of the RPR. When I took this test, my RPR (resting pulse rate) indicated thirty-six before the test; zero change for petro chemicals; but an eight point jump for formaldehyde.

OBSERVATION OF TEST RESULTS

From my observations because of the accuracy demonstrated by the CIRA test (close correlation to the intradermal test) I personally favor the CIRA test, followed up with a pulse test to confirm the offending foods.

Unfortunately, symptoms that seem to stem from food allergies might have a different cause. For instance, a yeast infection in the digestive tract may resemble a food allergy.

EXAMPLES OF SEVERE LIMITATIONS THAT SOME FOOD ALLERGIES CAN IMPOSE

Detailed here are three cases to show a sample of some of the drastic effects experienced from food allergies. Note the different ways these allergies become manifest.

Case A is Coca's wife. Angina pectoris came on her suddenly. Coca found potatoes to be the cause for her pulse to rise from 68 to 180! Through careful testing, he identified other food problems. These, too, were eliminated from her diet. In time she realized that other problems she thought to be a maternal inheritance did not recur, including migraines, colitis, and attacks of dizziness and fainting.

Case B comes from the preface of Coca's book. It relates a story about a man hospitalized without success for treatment of extremely painful and serious stomach ulcers, then cured in a matter of days after the discovery of his allergy to cow's milk; nutritious for most, but not for him. He continued to live an ulcer free life.

Case C is a story told in the March 31, 1985 issue of *The Parade Magazine* about Dr. Stuart Berger. At age nineteen, he weighed 420 pounds on a 6 foot 6.5 inch frame. All the diets he tried did not work. Even starving on 300 calories-a-day he failed to meet with success. *Wheat and dairy products* were eventually identified as the key culprits. Once these products were eliminated from his diet he readily lost his excess poundage. He finished Tufts University, leaving 200 pounds behind. He continued research into bariatics (the science of weight control) at Harvard.

More detail about my food allergies are made in Chapter 15, "So What Have I Learned."

By special permission, ARCO Publishing, New York.

Case A & B By special permission from ARCO Publishing, NY.

Case C By special permission from *The Parade Magazine*, copyright c 1985.

CHAPTER 6

Dental Health/Mercury Amalgams [Fillings]

My situation became desperate. The constant mental confusion, the short memory and the inability to concentrate caused considerable emotional distress. Dissatisfied with my job performance, I knew I had to shape up or put in for early retirement.

The thought of retirement held no appeal. Retiring would not fix my present mental state. However, it would save me from the embarrassment that comes from substandard performance.

Almost like a message from heaven, I received in the mail the *Gary Null Natural Living Newsletter* with articles about mercury amalgam poisoning. The letter advocated the removal of all mercury amalgams from one's mouth. Fortified with this information I came to the conclusion I should have all of mine removed; and I had a mouth full.

This occurred about the same time as the teeth cleaning and check up appointment. I asked my dentist about the mercury amalgam removal. He responded negatively at first. After about fifteen minutes of discussion, he relented but insisted the American Dental Association does not recognize the problem as one affecting very many people, only a limited few. Other dentists have reported in dental newsletters their patients who have had the removal done are most vociferous about the dramatic change in their health for the better.

Hal A. Huggins', D.D.S., book, *It's All in Your Head,* provides an in-depth discussion of the mercury amalgam problem.

He opens his book by briefly describing two specific cases to illustrate the danger of mercury amalgams.

- Case One is about a bright seventeen-year-old girl who had a bad experience after having three new fillings; she already had three before this episode. She suffered increasingly severe chest pains. More than fifty trips from one doctor to another failed to help. She had the full gamut of consultations with cardiologists and internists, and was hospitalized for detailed examinations with many specialists involved. All tests said "You're OK." Huggins described her as a "pimple faced, quivering pile of protoplasm trying to claw her heart out of her chest." Huggins removed the six small mercury amalgams and replaced them with plastic. Then good things started to happen. Two days later, the severe chest pains stopped. In four days she was again with her friends doing two semesters' work in one to graduate with them. Six small fillings made the difference between termination of life and graduation. A popular girl, a cheerleader and a bright and happy person, she went through the torments of hell because of mercury amalgams.

- Case Two—An eleven-year-old girl who had two small fillings done. Soon thereafter she started having seizures every fifteen minutes. Eight thousand dollars spent at a reputable hospital still did not isolate the problem. Doctors suggested she be put in an institution. This straight A student now could not walk or stand by herself, and could barely think. With fifteen minutes between seizures it became a real challenge for Huggins to remove the mercury amalgams since the removal/replacement process was interrupted by seizures. The dentist completed the elimination of the mercury amalgam on December 19th. By December 25th, this clear-headed young girl got out of bed, dressed and walked downstairs without assistance. What a Christmas present for the girl and Huggins! The seizures were completely eliminated. It is horrifying to think that two fillings came close to committing this person to a frightful life.

These cases make me wonder how many more individuals might be suffering needlessly. My case was not as severe, but at the same time it had a significant impact on my health and personality. Before detailing my personal experience, let me further expand on the danger of mercury amalgam.

Mercury is a poison. Specific instructions are given for the *safe handling* of mercury amalgam. Dentists are warned not to touch it with their bare hands. Yet this stuff is supposed to be safe in your mouth. This seems to be a contradiction.

Huggins explains that the mercury amalgam is fifty percent mercury when it is placed. Tests show this percentage is decreased with the age of the filling. Some tests indicate as low as five percent for twenty-year-old fillings.

By special permission from Dr. Huggins

In one patient, Huggins measured 90 mcg/m^3 vapor with a Bacarach Mercury Detector. The OSHA standard is 50 mcg/m^3. Consequently, this individual created his own health hazard on account of his mercury amalgam.

Huggins explained on page 29 of his book that chewing gum or food, smoking, or drinking alcohol sets up a varied environment causing the mercury to vaporize. This does harm to one or more of the body functions. Should the mercury vapor be compounded with a carbon-hydrogen compound of the methyl group, *methyl mercury results. This is 100 times more toxic than plain elemental mercury.* Methyl mercury is toxic to the nerve tissues and the brain. This may explain the relationship of the amalgam to epilepsy, multiple sclerosis or emotional problems.

The methyl mercury problem Huggins presents reminds me of a personal encounter. Years ago, while I sat at an army mess table, a young man sitting opposite me got up, lifted the table and turned it over. He fell writhing on the ground with an epileptic seizure. Could this have been from eating something that created the methyl mercury?

Huggins has seen many responses to mercury amalgam removal in six different categories as noted below. He goes on to explain the relationship and some case histories for each of them.

- neurological
- collagen
- allergy
- cardiovascular
- immunological
- miscellaneous

Are mercury fillings the only place where there is potential for mercury poisoning? The answer to this is surprising and frightening. Huggins' list almost fills three full pages (pages, 100, 101, 102).

I noticed that methyl mercury fungicides are used for treating seed grain. I had the job on the farm to put the fungicide dust on a pile of grain on the floor, and mix it with a scoop shovel; though I was warned not to breathe any of the dust, I had no mask for protection.

Other potential sources of problems that caught my eye include:

- hair dye
- mascara
- skin lightening creams
- toilet paper from recycled paper

Aside from the toxic effects already discussed, a second danger from fillings is electric currents. They raise abnormal responses in the neurological system. Huggins tells about a man who had a *tachycardia attack*. Tachycardia is described as a rapid heartbeat that starts and ends suddenly. It may last for minutes or days, giving a fluttering sensation in the chest.

Huggins states that it is important to understand what is in the mouth before mercury amalgam removal is done. Just removing or replacing fillings is a small part of the treatment for most people. New compatibility studies have demonstrated that some of the plastic fillings create immune system reactions in over fifty percent of the population. That's the frying pan into the fire syndrome. *You need to become self-educated before tackling the dental profession on a personal basis.* Huggins has a toll-free number so people can get the names of dentists who have been trained in the proper techniques. For your information it is 1-800-331-2303.

Huggins has developed the PAR (Proper Amalgam Removal) booklet to update you on his current findings. He receives a dozen calls a day from people who ran out and had their amalgams removed and are now "worse than they have ever been." Now we know why. Look over the PAR booklet and see how complex it is getting. We have advanced from Wright Brothers to 747 in the past ten years.

As if the mercury amalgam story is not bad enough, a substitute called copper amalgam is coming on the scene. This too should be avoided because of its cytotoxic qualities, according to Huggins.

Now, on to my personal experience. With 20–20 hindsight I can pinpoint the date when I started to act like a senile old man, immediately after I had a root canal on a molar. Lots of mercury. I had a poor memory, long and short term, and suffered with frequent bouts of mental confusion. For example, driving home on the same route I took daily, I would look around and not recognize anything, or remember my destination. My wife repeatedly scolded me for "acting like an old man." Her observation was correct, but I did not have any control over the situation. Having my mercury amalgam (silver fillings) replaced restored my mental health. To my amazement and pleasure I had a dramatic improvement which lasted.

Immediately after having my mercury amalgams replaced with composites, I stopped acting like an old man and noticed other changes for the better:

- Both long and short term memory improved; no more mental confusion.
- I became more assertive (not abrasive) in my relationships with other people, or groups of people. "Before" and "after" handwriting analyses tend to bear this out.
- I had, from my youth, a three to four second delay in responding in a normal conversation. Many times before I

started to talk I got an unsolicited prompting from the other party to *say something!*, either by verbal or visual message. That time lag was not just every now and then, but every time. I recall as a nine or ten year old, my elders repeatedly scolded me to "listen when somebody is talking to you." My response to a question was always—"What?" Since changing the fillings in my teeth both traits have vanished.

Again, with 20–20 hindsight, I can remember my dental hygiene habits were not good. I loved candy and other sweets. I brushed my teeth only once every week to ten days if the spirit moved me. As a consequence, I had several fillings before age nine, but, now all of that is behind me. It has been more than three years since I had the silver removed and I do not say "what?" any more. Also, I have no problem carrying on a normal conversation.

The "before" and "after" story of the mercury amalgam leaves me with the distinct impression of improved mental health. Additionally, I completely dismissed any thought of retirement. I can meet the requirements of my job with no difficulty.

As a matter of interest, my laboratory analysis revealed the following regarding mercury: 1.7 parts per million, which is less than the 2.5 parts per million considered acceptable. Still functional before the removal of mercury amalgam . . . but. . . .

What some people fail to recognize is that any amount of toxic metals in your body endangers your health. However, the medical world tends to compare a person's test against the *average*. And if that person's reading is *average* or under, he or she is supposedly safe. This is wrong. Any toxic metal, no matter how small the amount, should be dealt with as poison, especially when there is an option to use or not use mercury amalgams.

Incidentally, I have completed the basic course of chelation therapy which removes toxic metals from your body. At the outset of the therapy the mercury measured 1.2; and after twenty treatments .3 parts per million. I started chelation therapy more than two years after having the mercury amalgam replaced.

CHAPTER 7

Exercise

Exercise on a regular basis is important to maintain one's health. Exercise or the lack thereof has a direct relationship to weight control, energy level, and mental and physical health. The proper mental attitude has a lot to do with how "up" you feel about exercising.

In my adult life, I did not take exercise seriously until diagnosed as having cardiovascular disease, hardening of the arteries, at age 54. The doctor prescribed walking two miles, morning and evening, every day. As a result, my energy level and my health in general improved.

I thought I was doing quite well with my exercise program, until some years later when my dietician asked me how high my pulse rate rose when I walked. I answered "95 to 100." "That is not high enough," she said "You need to walk faster or jog to get your pulse up to at least 120." So I did. I started jogging at age 62. I got my pulse rate up to the 135 range with fantastic results. My resting pulse rate dropped to the 44 range after six months of daily jogging and my energy level increased significantly. Some further details of this are told under the heading of "Resting Pulse Rate" in Chapter 17.

Eventually, I worked up to jogging a solid three and one-half miles at a nine to ten minute per mile pace. I have run seven-and eight-minute miles, but not for more than one mile at a time.

I started experimenting with speed walking during some of my jogs. I really stretched it out. For a brief distance, I actually could speed walk faster than I jogged; approximately ten versus six mph, respectively. As luck would have it, I overdid the speed walking by stretching the stride too much. I either damaged a tendon or strained a muscle in my right knee which put a stop to my jogging and speed walking. The doctor says it may heal up in a year, or maybe never. So now I am relegated to the exercise bike. This I do four or five times a week for thirty to thirty-five minutes each time.

I also started walking up nine flights of stairs on a daily basis at age fifty-eight. However, I had to discontinue this at age sixty-four because of the knee problem.

About three years into my walking program, I started to think about the need to exercise my flabby upper body muscles. I started with push-ups. At first, I had a real struggle to do three. In my life, I cannot recall doing more than five or six push-ups at one time. Through persistence, I worked up to thirty-seven. I do thirty on a daily basis now. I also include some upper body exercises with ten pound weights.

When I used to get up in the morning and sit on the edge of the bed, my first thoughts were tired thoughts. So tired I did not feel like exercising. I would say to myself, "Gee, am I tired. I did not get a very restful sleep last night." It took me the longest time to recognize that my muscles, bones and nerves respond to my brain. I noticed I usually "got into gear" about one hour after I got to work. I became busy and forgot to "think tired." There is a truism: "you become what you think about most." My predominant thoughts used to be "thinking tired." "Tired" is no longer in my dictionary.

The following experience illustrates the extent of my new-found energy. Six months after I started jogging, and a long time after I stopped thinking tired, on a return trip from Florida, I got up at 3 a.m. and did thirty-six pushups, showered, got dressed and on the road by 3:30 a.m. I drove 500 miles to my home in about twelve hours, got into my jogging clothes and jogged four miles, a first for me. Back from jogging, I showered, fixed dinner, ate and cleaned up the dishes. Afterwards, I hung wallpaper for three hours and off to bed at

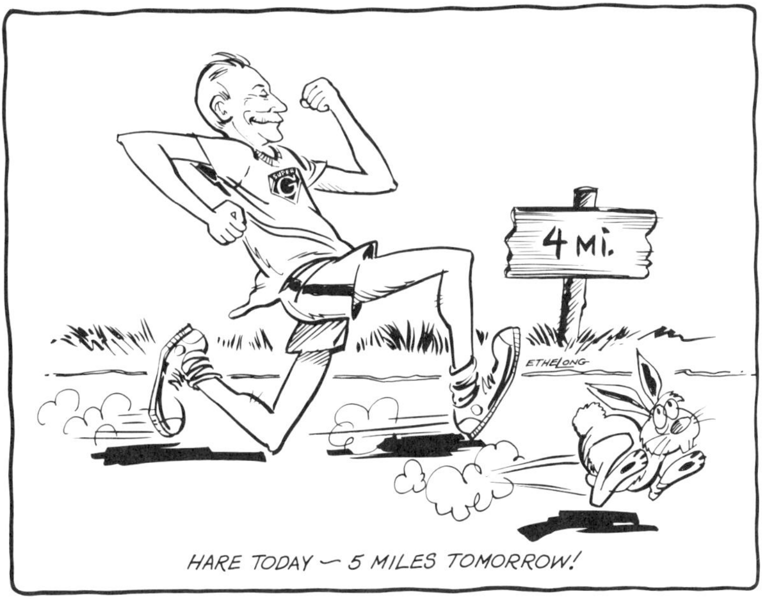

HARE TODAY — 5 MILES TOMORROW!

eleven p.m. The next day I got up at three a.m. and started wallpapering, but skipped the pushups. I wallpapered for twelve hours, stopping only briefly for breakfast and lunch. I then ironed twenty shirts while I watched the Super Bowl football game. Next I fixed dinner, ate, and cleaned the kitchen, then talked on the telephone with friends and relatives for about two hours. I will admit I did sleep very well the second night for six hours, then got up at five a.m. for a four-mile jog. I was not out to set an endurance record, but interested in continuing as long as I had the energy. I did this a week before my 63rd birthday. This abundance of energy is not an isolated case. The newfound energy is the reason I have become a fanatic about exercise. Besides improved energy level, weight control ceased to be a problem. The maintenance of my health is *priority one*—all other activities including work and play are the better for it.

CHAPTER 8

Chiropractic Treatment

As indicated in an earlier chapter, I was visiting Dr. J, a chiropractor, for guidance in the nutritional world. Office visits and time in the waiting room reading literature concerning chiropractic treatment raised my curiosity.

I did not have any problem with my back at the time. I hoped the examination would show something obvious to indicate potential connection with the dry mouth, but to no avail. My dry mouth greatly improved with vitamin supplements by the time I started chiropractic adjustments, but not 100 percent.

By the definition of chiropractors, given later in this chapter, Dr. J is a "mixer". Specifically, spinal manipulation, proper diet with appropriate vitamin and mineral supplements, and exercise are all a part of Dr. J's treatment program.

So I finally decided to proceed with the spinal manipulation. Pre-treatment x-ray examination revealed I had a slight curvature of the spine between my shoulder blades, explained as a "normal process of aging." Also, the x-ray showed a tightness between a couple of vertebrae in the neck and in the lower back, but no subluxations in evidence.

So now let me describe the treatment routine which proceeded as follows:

- I lay flat on my stomach on a padded treatment table while Dr. J examined my back with his fingers. He rapidly located one or more areas in my back where the muscle knotted. He massaged those areas with his fingers. This seemed to readily relieve the muscle tension. Also, he marked those spots with a felt-tipped pen for later application of the electronic massager.
- Next, traction was applied to the lower back to relieve spinal compressions and held for two to three minutes.
- For the "lumbar roll" I lay on my side with my upper leg in a slightly raised position. Then Dr. J put his knee on my leg to pin it down to the table. He then put his hands on my shoulder and pushed. This caused the back to twist or the "lumbar to roll" to keep the vertebrae from becoming fused. A popping similar to "cracking your knuckles" is the sign of success.
- Traction of the neck for two or three minutes was followed by a quick twist of the head in each direction, done while lying flat on my back.
- While I was sitting up on the edge of the examining table, Dr. J massaged the shoulder and neck muscles.
- He completed all of the manipulations in about fifteen minutes; then came the electronic massage.
- The electronic massage is a machine with one large paddle about the size of a ping pong paddle, and four smaller

ones resembling miniature ping pong paddles. The small paddles placed on the marked spots on my back. I lay face down, with the larger paddle placed under my abdomen. All the paddles had connecting wire to the control panel. Then the nurse placed a warm towel right up the middle of my back, a most pleasant sensation The more power applied to the electronic massager, the stronger the massage. The nurse set the timer for ten minutes.

I started out by taking one treatment a day for two weeks, followed by one treatment a week for about six months. Eventually these stretched to one every three months.

The results from the treatments follow:

- The stiffness of my back dissipated.
- The times I had to get up to go to the bathroom slacked off from seven or eight times every night down to one or two, and occasionally none.

Dr. J told me his mother-in-law suffered with colitis (ulcerated colon). The medication and treatment her medical doctor prescribed did not meet with the desired results. After some nagging Dr. J convinced her to have a spinal examination. This indicated a need for an adjustment. After three adjustments, her colitis cleared up.

While my improvement was not as spectacular as other people's such as Dr. J's mother-in-law, I was pleased with the results.

Let me explain what chiropractic is all about.

The reason I am including this information is because it addresses many of the same questions I asked myself regarding the benefits of chiropractic treatment.

The background regarding this subject is taken from the *1979 Chiropractic in New Zealand Report*. This report was written by a commission established by the command of His Excellency the Governor General of New Zealand; the commissioners:

- Brinsley Donald Inglis, c. B.A., J.D., L.L.D. chairman (B.A., Bachelor of Arts; J.D., Juris Doctor; L.L.D., Doctor of Laws)
- Betty Fraser, M.B.E., M.A. (M.B.E., Member of the order of the British Empire; M.A., Master of Arts)
- B. R. Penfold, M.Sc., PhD., F.R.S.N.Z. (M.Sc., Master of Science; Doctor of Philosophy; F.R.S.N.S., Fellow of the Royal Society [Science] of New Zealand

It is interesting the commissioners are not medical or chiropractic physicians.

However, the commission included a council comprised of representatives from the New Zealand Medical Association, the New Zealand Society of Physiotherapists, the New Zealand Chiropractors' Association, New Zealand Department of Health, and the New Zealand Consumer Council.

The commission was chartered to determine whether the New Zealand government should pay for chiropractic treatment under their Social Security Act and the Accident Compensation Act.

Specifically the Governor-general directed the commission to regard and consider:

- The practice and philosophy of chiropractic, its scientific and educational basis, and whether it constitutes a separate and distinct healing art

- The contribution chiropractic could make to the health services of New Zealand
- Any other matters considered relevant to the general objects of the inquiry.

The commission made inquiries in the United States where several of the New Zealand chiropractors received their training. The commission invited the medical association to present its own evidence, and to cross-examine any evidence presented on behalf of the chiropractic.

The commission's findings were unanimous. The general findings are presented below:

- Modern chiropractic is far from being an "unscientific cult."
- Chiropractic is a branch of the healing arts specializing in the correction by spinal manual therapy of what chiropractors identify as biomechanical disorders of the spinal column. They carry out spinal diagnosis and therapy at a sophisticated and refined level.
- Chiropractors are the only health practitioners equipped by their education and training to carry out spinal manual therapy.
- General medical practitioners and physiotherapists have no adequate training in spinal manual therapy, though a few have acquired skill in it subsequent to graduation.
- Spinal manual therapy in the hands of a registered chiropractor is safe.
- The education and training of a registered chiropractor is sufficient to enable him to determine whether there are contra-indications to spinal manual therapy in a particular case. He or she may also determine whether the patient should have medical care instead of or as well as chiropractic care.

- Spinal manual therapy can be effective in relieving musculo-skeletal symptoms such as back pain, and other symptoms known to respond to such therapy, such as migraine.
- In a limited number of cases where there are organic and/or visceral symptoms, chiropractic treatment may provide relief, but this is unpredictable, and in such cases the patient should be under concurrent medical care if practical.
- The precise nature of the biomechanical dysfunction which chiropractors claim to treat has not yet been demonstrated scientifically.

Additionally, the precise reasons why spinal manual therapy provides relief have not yet been scientifically explained. However, chiropractors have reasonable grounds based on clinical evidence for their belief that symptoms of the kind described above can respond beneficially to spinal manual therapy.

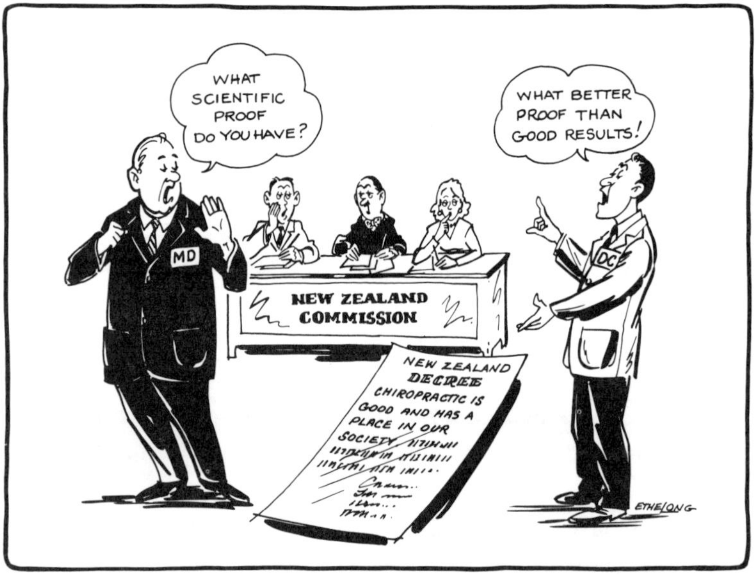
WHAT SCIENTIFIC PROOF DO YOU HAVE?
WHAT BETTER PROOF THAN GOOD RESULTS!
MD
DC
NEW ZEALAND COMMISSION
NEW ZEALAND DECREE
CHIROPRACTIC IS GOOD AND HAS A PLACE IN OUR SOCIETY
ETHELONG

Now a bit of history according to the New Zealand report. The earliest form of medical practice—"bonesetting" would now be described by the medical profession as manipulation, or the art of the chiropractic, often handed down in families. Mrs. Sarah Mapp learned the art from her father in the early 18th century. Sir Herbert Barker learned the art from his cousin. Sir Herbert was as well known in England as any doctor of his day (early 1900's) and recognized as the leading bonesetter. Good bonesetting resulted in significant relief in cases which defeated the efforts of the orthodox medical profession. Many of his successes were dramatic, but the forces of organized medicine fought him because of his lack of formal medical training. Nevertheless, Sir Herbert received the knighthood award in recognition of his services to public health.

The commission recognized that chiropractic started in the United States in the late 1800's. Dr. Andrew Taylor Sill, a country doctor from Virginia, became convinced the body cannot function properly unless it is structurally sound. If sound, the body's own recuperative powers will restore health. He developed a school of osteopathy in Kirksville, Missouri in 1882.

Daniel David Palmer established a second school in 1895. He cured his janitor of deafness by spinal manipulation. The janitor injured his back some seventeen years before, and from that time on he was nearly stone deaf. Palmer's success resulted from adjustments on the janitor to bring his vertebra back into alignment.

From the viewpoint of the New Zealand commission, osteopathy and chiropractic differences diminished with the years. Both arts appear to be the descendants of the bonesetter, but with the distinction that the art of the chiropractic has been developed and refined and taught to students with an aptitude for this art.

William Carver, an Oklahoma lawyer, established a school for the chiropractic in Oklahoma City. He believed chiropractic treatment in the adjustment of the spine by itself was not good enough. He believed in massage, heat therapy, and diet regulation. The Carver approach heralded the beginning of a split in the chiropractic world. The Chiropractors are now classified as:

- "mixers"—those who follow William Carver's precepts of including diet regulation, massage and heat therapy along with spinal adjustments.
- "straights"—those who confine themselves strictly to adjustments.

The New Zealand commission, because of the nature of its charter, confined its investigation to the efficacy of adjustments and all the ramifications of the chiropractic art related thereto. These are theory, education, advances in the art, and administration.

The theory of the chiropractic art is paraphrased below from the formal submissions to the commission by the New Zealand Chiropractic Association. This description is considered to address the central points of the chiropractic theory.

> "The practice of chiropractic has as its central therapeutic goal the restoration of normal function to the neuromusculoskeletal structures of the spine in order to advance the general welfare of the patient. Its focal point of concern is the integrity of the nervous system. The modern theory of chiropractic is no longer simple and direct nerve pressure, but is as complicated as the nervous system itself, with

recognition of the fact that the last word cannot be said in explanation for the success of chiropractic technique until the last words have been said in explanation of the complexities of the human nervous system. Chiropractors do not contend that subluxation, however defined, is the most significant causal factor in disease. They do claim that subluxations of different orders and types are a factor in the production of symptoms and that the adjustment of these subluxations brings about a return to more normal physiological functioning."

Chiropractic theory embraces both the Type M and Type O disorders.

- Type M are musculo-skeletal disorders involving basically a mechanical dysfunction. The symptoms are mainly a local pain in the spine or associated areas, such as a simple backache or headache.
- Type O involves organic or visceral disorders, such as high blood pressure, colitis, peptic ulcer. The claim of healing Type O disorders by spinal manipulation is a point with which the medical profession is in sharp disagreement.

The Chiropractors' Association in its formal submissions says "although mechanical malfunction of the spinal column is not claimed to be the most significant causal factor in disease, it is claimed to be a factor in the production of symptoms and that its correction brings about a return to more normal functioning."

This is of course a generalized and unspecific way of rationalizing the relief of Type O disorders which can sometimes be achieved by a chiropractor's treatment. But it carries important implications. For if a spinal mechanical malfunction is found to exist in any particular case, then its correction must, at the very least, according to the chiropractor, remove an impediment to the natural working of the body's system. This enables the body's natural defense mechanism against disorder and disease to operate more effectively and without that impediment. That naturally does not exclude the possibility that chiropractic treatment can work in a more direct manner, but in a way that cannot for the present be scientifically explained, to relieve some cases of Type O disorder.

"Further," according to the commission, "the concept of the vertebral subluxation is central to chiropractic." It postulates the existence of a class of spinal abnormalities which the chiropractor believes contributes to pain and other bodily disturbances. He seeks to identify such an abnormality and will direct his manual therapy toward attempting to correct it. He regards such an abnormality as causing various kinds of interference within the nervous system. That interference in his view can cause local pain, or it may be a factor in producing other disorders."

The concept of the subluxation is not inherently a complicated one, and the essential elements are clear . . .

- Abnormal function in a spinal joint.
- Neurological involvement.
- Perhaps, but not necessarily, displacement of a vertebra.

The commission goes on to say the problem is a functional not a structural one . . . The abnormal function of the spine may produce a vascular involvement as well as the neurological one, and this vascular involvement, originally emphasized in osteopathy, is now accepted by chiropractors generally.

The detection of the subluxation is a skill possessed only by the chiropractor. He will palpate the spinal column in order to detect areas of tenderness, abnormal function, or spinal deviation, but palpation alone will not determine the presence of a subluxation. The chiropractor will also evaluate the posture of the patient and take a case history. He will take an X-ray, not for the purpose of diagnosing the subluxation, but in order to exclude pathologies and contra-indications to manipulation. It is a combination of these factors which enables the chiropractor to say that a subluxation is present.

The New Zealand report explores in great detail the objections to the chiropractic by the medical profession. Simply stated, the medical profession believes chiropractic theory has no scientific basis to support its claims. Nonetheless, the chiropractic art has made significant contributions to the maintenance of one's health by spinal manipulation. Those interested in further exploring this argument may find The New Zealand report available from the Palmer College of Chiropractic, 1000 Brady Street, Davenport, Iowa 52803; cost $9.00 plus postage.

The case of Mr. T is presented as an example of chiropractic treatment. The details of this case are presented on pages 174 and 175 of the *Report on the Chiropractic in New Zealand.* Mr. T. was severely injured in an automobile accident and paralyzed from his waist down, losing his sense of balance and coordination. Specialists in the hospital could not improve his condition and told him he would have to "learn to live with his problem." On a friend's recommendation, he tried chiropractic treatment. He took his first steps after six months, and went back to normal after twelve months. The problem involved "severe locking" of the fourth and fifth lumbar, clearly visible on the x-rays.

I am impressed that chiropractic treatment is good. If I get some ailment in the future that fails to respond to treatment, I will have a chiropractor examine my back to eliminate it as a probable cause. The condition of subluxation in your spine can raise havoc with your health. Normal, conventional treatments by doctors will be to no avail until the subluxation is corrected. The chiropractor is the skilled health professional to accomplish this task.

I believe it is good to visit a chiropractor on a periodic basis to keep your spine in proper alignment.

CHAPTER 9

Health Profile Update

There are two reasons for this update. First, I want the reader to know of my progress in maintaining a state of *wellness*. I am pleased with myself insofar as the original list is concerned. I considered my health to be under control; and the occurrence of new problems would be held to a minimum. So much for that happy thought; five new problems arrived.

The second reason for the update is to establish a "before health condition" immediately prior to the chelation therapy presented in Chapter 10. So now on to the details of:

- recap of continuing problems
- summary of new problems
- diet and exercise regimen

Recap of continuing problems before chelation therapy:

- dry mouth—some problems although I got along without artificial saliva, my mouth was not totally recovered. There continued to be short periods of dryness.
- hardening of the arteries—still present, more symptoms, ie. frequent dizziness, slurred speech, and a numb foot. This is the primary reason for taking chelation therapy.

Summary of new problems appearing in the intervening three and one-half year period:

- malabsorption—a digestive system dysfunction; this subject is treated in detail in Chapter 12.
- short term memory and ability to concentrate in a decline. However, this situation disappeared with the removal of my mercury amalgam fillings.
- poor leg muscle strength below the knee—my legs felt like lead when I walked and jogged.
- xerosis—a patch of dry skin on my buttocks that would not respond to prescription drugs (ointments) or diet.
- resting pulse rate (RPR)—My RPR registered around 44 most of the time, presumably because of my exercise program. However, it drifted to as low as 36 beats per minute; normal for most people is 60 to 75.

Now to recap the numbers before starting chelation therapy:

- from the Chapter 3 tabulation, two of twenty-three items not fully resolved.
- five new difficulties identified.
- total of seven dysfunctions to grapple with.

Diet and exercise regimen. I altered my diet to comply with the food allergy tests. However, I slacked up in maintaining my diet at the three year point. There are more details on this in the food allergy chapter. The exercise program went from walking to jogging and speed walking, then on to the exercise bike, upper body exercise added; also push-ups and weight lifting.

CHAPTER 10

Chelation Therapy

By this time I realized some success in overcoming the dry mouth and dry eye condition. In the process, many health improvements were holding up.

I decided to watch my diet, do the vitamin and mineral supplementation, exercise regularly and grow old gracefully. But life is full of the unexpected.

I became aware of a numb foot; I felt light-headed many times a day, everyday; and troubled frequently with slurred speech. The first item clearly an indication of poor circulation, the other two are characteristic of an impending stroke. I must tell you I am greatly afraid of strokes and snakes. Consequently, it motivated me to take action to eliminate the problem of a potential stroke. I already knew how to take care of snakes—just keep out of their way.

Gary Null's *Natural Living Newsletter* first brought Chelation Therapy to my attention. Better take the treatment I thought, better to be safe than sorry.

There are several parts of this to be told to give you a coherent story. In the following order I will tell about:

- The "what" and "how" of chelation therapy.
- The chelation formula used.
- Action and reactions to the treatment.
- A summary of the physical and mental changes noted.
- A brief summary of a number of other cases, most of which are fellow patients.
- The magic of chelation therapy.

The "what" and "how" of chelation therapy. The following is based on information published by the American Academy for Medical Preventics, now the American College for the Advancement in Medicine. Chelation therapy involves the intravenous feeding of a chemical commonly referred to as EDTA ***(ethylene diamine tetra acetate)***. EDTA has a single unique characteristic of attaching to toxic metals and some minerals. Once the EDTA binds together with the metal and/or calcium buildup in the arteries, it is excreted through the urine. The toxic minerals list includes arsenic, lead, mercury and aluminum.

In clogged arteries, the inner surface includes a plaque containing some calcium. The EDTA removes the calcium thereby restoring a more normal blood flow. An increase in diameter of a diseased artery of as little as ten to twenty percent is sufficient to approximately double the flow of blood. Before serious symptoms of a heart disease become apparent the occlusion of the artery is in the vicinity of 85 percent.

The EDTA therapy session, which takes about three hours, is done on an outpatient basis. Twenty-five to thirty treatments are a normal base course depending on the problem being addressed. The 1989 cost per treatment typically is in the $85 to $100 range. Thus the $3,000 for chelation therapy compares with the $35,000 to $40,000 for arterial bypass operations.

Chelation therapy has been used in the treatment of occlusive arterial disease for more than twenty years and reported on extensively in the peer review scientific literature.

The American Board of Chelation Therapy provides a training and certification program.

The American College for the Advancement in Medicine (ACAM) is a professional association of physicians who practice advanced medicine and have a special interest in chelation therapy. The ACAM maintains and promulgates a protocol of professionally recognized standards of practice for the safe and effective administration of intravenous EDTA chelation therapy in the treatment of age associated diseases, including atherosclerotic vascular disease. According to the ACAM literature, there has not been one recorded death as a result of chelation therapy using the protocol they have established.

James J. Julian, M.D., author of *Pass or Bypass (Chelation Extends Life),* dedicated his book "to all those who don't want to wait for a stroke, heart attack, or senility to qualify them for health care." Julian advises that *the need for chelation therapy is related to the deposition of toxic metals and/or the conditions of the arteries and not age per se.* He states that eighty percent of the autopsied American soldiers from the Korean and Vietnam Wars showed advanced atherosclerosis (hardening of the arteries). Whereas the enemy soldiers autopsied showed little atherosclerosis. This relationship obviously existed because of different diets.

Four areas of the cardiovascular system that are frequent blockage sites:

- arteries to the head, and in the head
- arteries associated near the heart
- arteries in the lower back area
- arteries in the knees

Julian presented a case history of a 72-year old man with seven blockages diagnosed by an angiogram.

- 97 percent blockage of the main anterior descending artery
- two areas blocked by 90 percent
- two more areas blocked at 85 percent
- one at 75 percent; and
- one at 65 percent

Incidentally this patient, a medical doctor, chose chelation therapy over bypass surgery. He returned to an active lifestyle after completing the course of chelation therapy.

Chelation therapy began as treatment for lead poisoning. This therapy, when applied to adults, resulted in improvements beyond what could be expected from just lead removal. The chelation therapy not only removed the lead, it also unblocked arteries to promote other improvements. This included diminished leg and heart pains, improved memory, better eyesight and other health benefits.

Chelation therapy is approved by the United States Food and Drug Administration for hypercalcemia (high blood calcium levels), for chelating heavy metals (lead, mercury, arsenic, aluminum), and for toxicity from the drug digitalis.

By special permission from D. J. J. Julian.

To find a physician who is trained and competent to administer chelation therapy contact:

American College of Advancement in Medicine
23121 Verdugo Drive Suite 204
Laguna Hills, California 92653
Telephone (714) 583-7666

The Chelation Formula—The differences are in the time it takes to administer, normally about three hours: and whether it is full strength, one-half or one-quarter strength depending on the health of the patient. I take the full strength administered in the normal time, at about one drop per second.

500 ml sterile water add
20 ml EDTA (Ethylene diamine tetera acetate)
30 ml ascorbic acid (vitamin C)
10 ml magnesium chloride
5 ml lidocaine
5 ml potassium chloride
2 ml folic acid
0.6 ml heparin
2 ml B complex vitamin

Action and reaction to the treatment— This addresses the physical reaction to the therapy, not the results thereof. The reactions are noted below:

- During the IV (intravenous) feeding
  + ache in the same arm as the IV needle, most of the time the pain was very small; sometimes moderately painful. This would come and go at random.
  + my face would feel slightly flushed a few times during the feeding, but only for brief periods.

  + In my first session, a feeling of nausea came on after about one and one-half hours. A snack brought instant relief. So now, as a matter of practice, I have a snack after about one hour of IV.
- After the IV feeding
  + feel a bit woozy initially upon standing up after treatment. This feeling dissipates in less than one minute.
  + a dry mouth comes on typically for me about two hours after the treatment. This condition lasted about twenty-four hours before returning to normal.

Summary of changes noted from the IV chelation therapy:

- dry mouth—some problems continue, more about this later in Chapter 16. After twenty-two treatments there was no apparent change in the dry mouth.
- hardening of the arteries—this means poor circulation, confirmed by a Therma-Scan test described in Chapter 13. After fifteen treatments, the light-headedness disappeared. However, the foot numbness did not fade away completely until after twenty-eight chelation therapy sessions.
- leg muscle strength below the knee felt like lead. As a matter of fact, for years I scuffed my feet as I walked, which is hard on the heels of my shoes. After four treatments I no longer scuffed my heels when I walked.
- xerosis—responded to the chelation therapy. After four treatments, the xerosis was completely gone. No drugs or ointments were used in conjunction with the chelation therapy. Xerosis is an abnormally dry area of the skin. In my case, it was on my rump and it itched now and then.
- resting pulse rate—Four doctors had no explanation why my pulse rate would drift to 36, from 44 to 46; or if it were a warning of a further breakdown of my health. My intuition told me something was wrong and something worse about to happen. After ten chelation therapy ses-

sions my RPR does not drift; *and* raised to the 52–54 range.

- cosmetic changes—The changes noted help me to look younger, and to feel younger and more alive. This is my assessment:
  + My skin, all over my body looks healthier. The appearance and feel of my face is healthier. The skin of my legs and under my arms is no longer pale white, like bleached flour, but almost like a light suntan.
  + The sparkle in my eyes came back soon after I started my allergy diet, but now I have a *super sparkle.*
  + The color of my hair reversed from nearly all gray back to blond on the top of my head. The "white side walls" have yet to show any change.
  + The hair on my legs returned in full strength, an amazing sight to me. For years my leg hair resembled a molting chicken. The healthy skin and stand of hair give my legs a younger look. When I wear shorts a lady friend compliments me on my "sexy legs."
  + The depth of the wrinkles at the corner of my eyes significantly diminished, almost to the point of looking like a face lift.

Summary of fellow chelation patients' experiences: Most of these cases are spectacular compared to my experience.

At the beginning of my first treatment I started to read a book entitled *Bypassing the Bypass* by Dr. Cranton. Astounded as I browsed through the book, I read aloud. The book claimed chelation therapy improved eyesight. I said, "How could this be. Is it really true?" I got an instant reply from a fellow patient, a 75-year-old-man—"Positively yes is the answer, my eyesight is definitely improved!"

Now on to experiences of patients with whom I had personal contact during my treatment.

- *Case A* a woman in her mid-50s. Her health condition immediately prior to the starting of chelation therapy was classified as desperate. The opthamologist's prognosis—totally blind in less than six months because he could see the blood vessels in her eyes were drying up. Intolerant of medication to control her high blood pressure, 240/130. A cholesterol count in the 500s. She barely could walk from her bed to the bathroom. After thirty treatments, the eyesight restored, blood pressure 130/80 without the benefit of drugs; cholesterol count near normal; and she was up and about doing the things healthy people do.
- *Case B* a stroke victim about age 45. As I started my second treatment, they wheeled him in for his first. Paralyzed down his right side, he could not move his right arm or his right leg. After three treatments, he was able to stand up. A few treatments later, he could take a few steps with a walker. Soon he walked with the aid of a cane. He is taking physical therapy along with chelation therapy. His outlook is for continued improvement.
- *Case C* a woman, in her late 40s. Before starting her chelation therapy, she was diagnosed as having multiple sclerosis (MS). The medication did nothing positive for her. She learned of chelation therapy and decided to give it a try. When she went to the chelation doctor she had a battery of lab tests done. He told her he could not confirm she had MS, but he could confirm that she had a high count of aluminum, which is poisonous to the body. Her count of thirty compared to an average of six to fourteen. Her left foot dragged as she walked, and her right eye gave her trouble. After about thirty treatments, she was back to normal, her "MS" overcome.

So, you may ask, where does a person pick up aluminum? Consider the following list of potential contributors:

- underarm deodorants
- antacid tablets
- non-dairy creamers
- public drinking water—aluminum oxide is used to take the cloudiness out of the water.
- cookware
- beer and pop cans
- baking powder

• *Cases D, E, and F* are all the same. These are men of ages 35 to 51. They were all there to avoid bypass surgery. D got his maintenance treatment, once every three months. The others were there because they, too, wanted to avoid bypass surgery and they knew of D. E, after eight treatments, said his chest pains were not as frequent or as severe as in the past and he felt strong enough to go back to work. But let me tell you a little more about D. He was forty-seven years old when one day he passed out on the kitchen floor. The doctor advised him he needed immediate bypass surgery; the sooner the better. D hesitated. He said he wanted to check with his family doctor to learn what the alternatives might be. Besides, D could not afford the $30,000 bill for heart surgery. His family doctor advised him to try chelation therapy. After thirty treatments, D restored to normal health and he was able to go back to work. D noted his hair color changed from graying, back to black.

• *Case G*—This man about 50 years old was the husband of C. G suffered from unexplained back problems. In spite of many medical examinations and chiropractic treatments, the problem went unresolved for more than 10 years. The pain became so severe it limited his physical activities. He could not do such simple things as yardwork or wash the car. With the discovery of his wife's problem of excessive aluminum content in her body, he decided to get a checkup. His lab test also revealed an abnormal count of aluminum. After chelation therapy, the miseries with his back disappeared. If there is a lesson here, it is that the effects (symptoms) relating to aluminum are not always the same. Some other cases I know of tend to bear this out.

- *Case H*—a man in his mid-70s who suffered a stroke. As a result, he had difficulty with his speech, double vision, and a big toe that turned black before the stroke, indicative of a circulatory problem. The stroke confirmed he did have a circulatory problem. With chelation therapy, his speech and double vision problems were eliminated, and his black toe returned to a normal, healthy color in the process.
- This case is not an individual one. I witnessed a videotape presentation by a doctor who used chelation therapy to treat five people with skin ulcers two to three inches in diameter, generally around the calf muscle, except for one individual who had a series of ulcers on both feet. The videotape showed pictures of the ulcers at various stages of the chelation therapy. In all cases but one, the ulcers healed, and the skin grew back. However, all of them had failed to respond to antibiotic treatment. In one case the large ulcer dried up but the skin did not grow back.

The magic of chelation therapy—The chelation improves blood circulation to all parts of the body, allowing the organs, lymph glands and all other parts of the body's chemical factory to get back to a more normal functioning. Additionally, the treatment eliminates (chelates) the toxic metals from your body, thus relieving the neurological system from needless stress. Then the body's immune system takes over and the miracles begin to happen. What other explanation can there be?

A significant problem with chelation therapy is that it sounds like a fairy tale since it seems to correct so many health problems. True to the American belief—"if it is too good to be true, it probably is not true." One of the cautions on a U.S. Department of Health and Human Services brochure on "Quackery" states: "Beware of a single product or treatment effective for a wide variety of ailments."

If the above listing of significant successes from chelation therapy were examined from the singular event of restoration of the circulatory system, then it does not appear to be a fairy tale. A corollary would be like aspirin affecting the neurological system, yielding relief to a number of symptoms such as with colds, headaches, aching joints, arthritis pain, etc.

CHAPTER 11

Vitamin and Mineral Supplementation

It is impossible to buy milk that is not fortified with Vitamin D. As a matter of fact, Vitamin D is found as an additive in most cereals, flour, and breads. Additionally, Vitamin D is the sunshine vitamin absorbed through the skin. On the vitamin shelf of the drug store, you'll find calcium fortified with Vitamin D, sixty percent of the recommended daily allowance. Consider this:

- Vitamin D aids in the absorption of calcium according to an article titled "Some Facts and Myths of Vitamins," Public Health Service, Food and Drug Administration. This is the good news.
- The presence of high blood levels of Vitamin D_2, used to fortify milk, encourages calcium deposition along artery walls. This the bad news. *Pass or Bypass,* James J. Julian, M.D., page 33.
- Excess Vitamin D intake blocks calcium absorption.

Now consider the person who drinks no more than one gallon of milk per week, daily gets approximately sixty percent RDA (recommended daily allowance) requirements of Vitamin D from this source. Couple this with a daily supplement of calcium fortified by Vitamin D; another sixty percent and with the added Vitamin D from breads, cereals and sunshine and the intake is well above 100 percent which will block calcium absorption.

Garry F. Gordon, D., M.D. says in *New Dimensions in Calcium Metabolism* that excess Vitamin D is a primary causitive factor among our population suffering with a deficiency leading to osteoporosis.

My comments on this situation are:

- The persistent efforts by the food industry to fortify products with various vitamins and minerals messes up Mother Nature.
- There are claims and counterclaims galore concerning vitamins. The question is, whom do you believe?
- Vitamin and/or mineral supplementation to your diet should be taken only after the advice and guidance of a dietitian or nutritionist.

I am going to address my vitamin *and mineral* supplementation later in this chapter. But, before I get into those details, I want to tell about the hair test to determine nutrient mineral levels and toxic mineral levels.

The technical information regarding hair testing is taken from my Mineral Analysis Report by Doctor's Data. Minerals are stored in various parts of the body such as the liver, brain, muscles, heart, skin and hair. Scientists have learned that the hair on the nape of your neck contains representative levels of nutrient and toxic minerals.

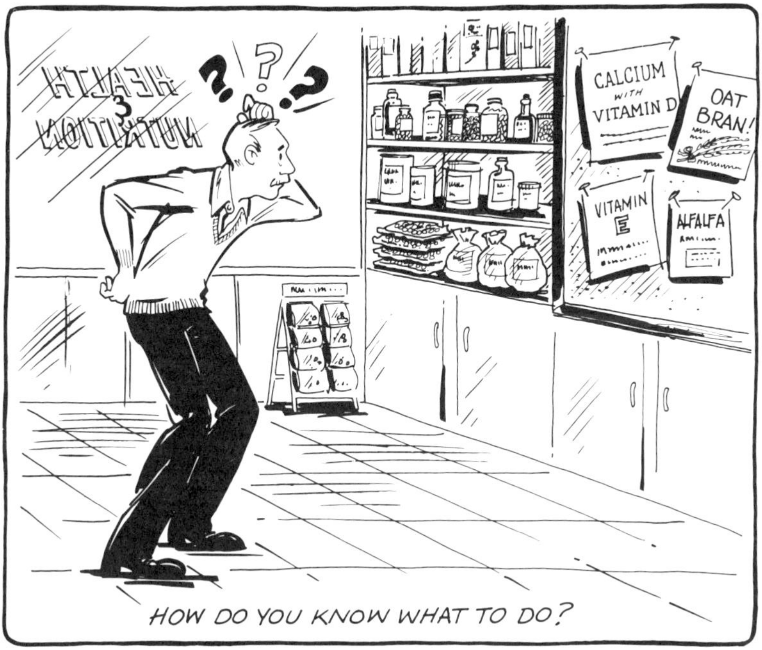

After a hair sample is taken, it is cleaned and given a spectographic analysis. The accuracy of the analysis is dependent on the procedures established and followed by the lab technicians who processes the sample. Reliable results depend upon receipt of a good specimen. Bleached, dyed, or permed hair is not acceptable. The results from the hair tests are repeatable.

The essential biological organic nutrients are called vitamins, amino and fatty acids. The essential minerals are the other part of this chemical puzzle needed to maintain your health.

Doctor's Data explains that the test identifies the toxic mineral levels. Some toxic minerals are needed at extremely low levels. However it is common to exceed the healthy amount, and at the higher levels they become toxic. Any mineral can become toxic at a high enough level. The higher the level, the more toxic the reaction that can cause sickness or death.

The results of the tests are given in finite numbers against the reference range for the mineral levels. The reference range is established by statistical logarithmic average of a healthy population. The reference range is described as one standard deviation above and below the mean; this represents about 68 percent of the selected healthy population. Two standard deviations include 95 percent of the selected healthy population.

Figure 11-1 depicts the results of four tests I have taken during the first four years of my health program.

MINERAL & METAL LEVELS

Minerals	Age	62 11/85	63 3/86	63 6/86	64 3/87	Reference Range
*Calcium		151	262	160	151	325–934
*Magnesium		13	25	9	10	32–122
Sodium		53	162	40	82	27–163
Potassium		19	39	13	13	11–80
*Copper		7	7	7	8	11–41
Zinc		152	154	124	137	124–184
*Iron		6	5	5	4	5–18
*Manganese		.12	.17	.19	.09	.27–1.54
*Chromium		.57	.80	.36	.42	.61–1.39
*Cobalt		.22	.12	.08	.07	.12–.31
Lithium		.014	.119	.040	.078	.006–.427
Molybdenum		1.25	1.64	.80	.90	.20–1.43
Phosphorus		143	134	114	130	108–178
Selenium		.5	.2	.2	.3	.16–.88
*Silicon		6	3	3	2	4–11
Vanadium		.10	—	.11	.16	.08–.25

*Below Normal

FIGURE 11–1

If nutrient mineral levels are predominantly low, malabsorption should be suspected. The same is true if calcium, magnesium and zinc levels are more than one standard above the mean. (Note: there are different opinions on this.)

In my case, the nutrient levels are indeed predominantly low with 10 of the 15 minerals examined below one standard deviation.

The toxic mineral levels are shown in Figure 11–2. The March 87 level of aluminum is two against thirty as one standard deviation above the mean. The blood serum test taken at the same time had a count of ten against an average range of six to fourteen. This is not an apples and apples test. On one hand the hair test indicates the tissue mineral level; the blood serum test indicates just that—the mineral level in the blood.

Doctor's Data goes on to explain that high toxic mineral levels contribute to impaired function of cell metabolism. This also may cause interference with absorption of nutrient

TOXIC METAL LEVELS

					One Standard Deviation
Lead	1	4	2	1	15
Arsenic	.6	2.2	.3	.4	7.0
Mercury	1.7	2.9	.7	1.2	2.5
Cadmium	.4	.3	.3	.2	1.0
Aluminum	2	3	1	2	30.0
Nickel	1.2	.6	.5	.3	2.2
Beryllium	.027	.022	.008	.008	.1

FIGURE 11–2

minerals. Low levels of nutrient minerals may contribute to the absorption of the toxic minerals—an unwanted happening. Conversely, a healthy level of nutrient minerals tends to block the absorption of toxic metals. Examination of my mineral levels indicates I am vulnerable to the absorption of the toxic metals because of my low levels of nutrient minerals.

The history of my vitamin and mineral supplementation after I started eating to live four years ago is presented in Figure 11–3. Prior to this time I indulged in one-a-day vitamins off and on; zinc on a consistent basis for the past 10 years (six years prior to eating to live plus four years); iron tablets on a sporadic basis without any apparent success. My tests showed no improvement in the clinical measure of my iron—always marginal anemia. This is true with the exception of the one blood test taken about four months after I started my health attack; maybe an accurate measurement, maybe not. I learned Vitamin C aids in the absorption of iron.

Some of the highlights of observations and commentary to the hair test made by the laboratory are presented below by each significant deficiency noted as abnormal. The personal

VITAMIN AND MINERAL SUPPLEMENTATION

SUPPLEMENTS	1983	1984	1985	1986	1987
Multivitamin	X	X	X	X	X
B Complex	X	X	X		X
Vitamin C	X	X			
Calcium	X	X	X		X
Iron		X	X		
Zinc	X	X	X	X	X
Amino Acids	X	X	X		

FIGURE 11–3

measurements in these tests are taken from the March 1987 report. This was at the beginning of the chelation therapy.

Head hair *calcium* less than 325 parts per million (PPM); my level measured at 151 more than three standard deviations low, really low. Doctor's Data explains that depressed calcium affects many systems of the body and therefore insufficient calcium can be expected to affect many aspects of the human system. Abnormalities in calcium tissue levels occur frequently and are often difficult to manage.

Obvious symptoms of depressed calcium levels are noted below; however, most often no direct clinical symptoms are noticed.

- *muscle cramps
- *brittle fingernails
- periodontal conditions (long-term deficiency)
- osteoporosis (long-term deficiency)
- *gray or white hair reflect approximately 30 percent lower calcium levels

FOOTNOTE: *indicate symptoms applying to me.

Causes of low calcium are:

- insufficient or excess phosphorus
- insufficient or excess vitamin D-3
- insufficient magnesium
- hyperthyroidism
- alcoholism
- elevated toxins

Head hair *magnesium* deficiency less than 32 PPM; my level was measured at 10 PPM, more than three standard deviations on the low side.

My lab report from Doctor's Data stated that hair magnesium levels can be a more sensitive indicator than either blood or urine tests. Magnesium is involved in over 75% of all enzyme functions. Insufficient magnesium can result in various clinical conditions but usually result in subclinical or non-clinical conditions.

The symptoms for depressed magnesium levels are presented below, but not usually seen unless levels are below two standard deviations:

- *depression
- *muscle tension
- irritability, nervousness, hypertension
- *hyperactivity

The causes for insufficient magnesium levels are:

- insufficient ingestion of magnesium
- exposure to toxic metals
- alcoholism
- depression
- hypothyroidism

Head hair *copper* deficiency less than 11 PPM: my level measured at 8 PPM, more than one standard deviation on the low side.

Copper is involved in several enzyme functions, and therefore involved with various aspects of the body. Copper and iron are required for normal metochondrial electron transport and other cellular energy functions. Copper is also required as a precursor of iron in the formation of hemoglobin and to convert T4 to T3. Copper is a part of the MAO regulatory functions of the brain.

These symptoms are often observed when copper is below two standard deviations.

- *thyroid malfunction
- *zinc imbalance

Copper deficiency is associated with:

- elevated serum cholesterol due to reduced bile functions
- elevated levels of molybdenum

Head hair *zinc* less than 124 PPM; my level measured at 124 PPM, less than one standard deviation on the low side. At one standard deviation below the reference range, one or more of the following symptoms may occur:

- loss of taste sensitivity is commonly the first symptom to be observed. This causes the increased use of salt and spices
- vitamin A non-responsive night blindness
- *white spots on finger nails
- delayed wound healing

Significant zinc depression, below two standard deviations, could produce the following:

- impaired growth function
- impaired T4 to T3 conversion
- dysmenorrhea
- *underdeveloped primary and secondary sex characteristics including sperm count

The usual causes of zinc depression are typically:

- lack of zinc availability in the the diet
- excessive alcohol consumption

- in males, a very active sex life
- stress
- elevated toxic metals
- excess of copper assimilation

Head hair *iron* less than 5 PPM; my level measured at 4, just slightly more than one standard deviation low.

Head hair iron tests do not necessarily correlate with blood serum tests. Low hair levels of iron may indicate a deficiency months before it is detected in the blood. However, hair and tissue levels of iron do have a close match.

Iron deficiency symptoms include:

- breathing difficulties
- *brittle nails
- pale skin
- fatigue
- constipation
- sore or inflamed tongue

Causes for iron deficiencies are:

- diets high in phyates
- diets high in oxylates
- diets high in phosphates
- insufficient iron ingestion
- excess tea, zinc or copper

Head hair tests showing combination low levels of calcium, magnesium, zinc and chromium often have been observed with the individual who has been exposed to stress or toxins. When the stress or toxins have been removed, these minerals will approach the reference range.

With head hear zinc less than 130 PPM in combination with copper less than 12 PPM, it has been observed there is a higher experience of hypothyroidism.

Doctor's Data explains that with head hair copper less than 11: with zinc less than 124; and iron less than 5 in combination, the individual will show insufficient stomach acid (pH). The absorption of a number of minerals is sensitive to the pH of the stomach (calcium, magnesium, copper, zinc, manganese and chromium).

The end of the laboratory's report stated: "No significant elevation of any one of the toxic metals was found at this time." Some of the common factors in reducing toxins are: chelation, reduced toxic exposure, ingestion of vitamin C, and high levels of amino acids of the sulphydryl groups (March 1987 hair test).

My commentary on the above hair tests is that malabsorption is the basic problem. This has continued to be my problem even with taking supplements. However, it is early September 1987, as I write this, and I have been taking hydrochloric acid tablets (Betain) since March 1987 as a means to provide pH to aid in the digestive process. I hoped I would see some improvement in my next hair test. But, I was in for a surprise. The details are covered in Chapter 12, "Malabsorption."

By special permission from Doctor's Data.

CHAPTER 12

Malabsorption

Malabsorption came to light when I started taking vitamin and mineral supplements. The pills I swallowed went through my system but did not fully digest. They repeatedly showed up in my stools. This hint of malabsorption was confirmed by subsequent lab tests.

My dietitian reasoned the malabsorption process was caused by a lack of hydrochloric acid being generated by my system. Consequently, I started taking Betaine tablets as a crutch. The trade name of the tablets is Hydro-Zyme, Biotics Research Corp., Houston, Texas. The tablets contain Betaine HCL, pepsin, ammonium chloride, glutamic acid HCL, vitamin B-6 and pancreatin 4X. Pancreatin (4X) is coated for release in the intestinal tract and for protection from the acidic stomach environment.

The first few days I took this it gave me a feeling of euphoria. I thought this resulted from getting more nutrients absorbed from my foods. This happy feeling soon wore off. Malabsorption continued to be confirmed by poor readings on the mineral levels from the hair analyses. I am still grappling with the malabsorption dysfunction.

My continued investigation into this condition led me to the gastrogram test. This test reveals the pH (acidity) of the stomach and small intestine. My stomach and small intestine turned out to have below normal pH, and the transit time through the stomach was too slow.

The normal pH of the small intestine is neutral 7.0 to alkaline 9.0. Liver bile and pancreatin from the pancreas need this neutral to alkaline condition to work properly to break down fats and convert proteins to amino acids.

The amino acids are the fundamental building blocks of life—therefore, it is important for your doctor to know the pH of your stomach and small intestine.

My lab report from the gastrogram test indicated that the hyperacidity (low pH) and delayed emptying times often result in malabsorption, stomach gas, bloating, belching and flatulence. Although I am somewhat improved from prior years I still have not overcome malabsorption.

What follows is the gastrogram results from my test and the prescribed therapy.

- The stomach acid level is too high.
- The stomach emptying time into the small intestine is too slow. This indicates that foods are being overly prepared for digestion before it reaches the small intestine. Delayed

emptying time destroys much of the nutrient value of the foods.

- The small intestine's pH range is suboptimal at 5.5.

The initial therapy prescribed is to:

- Take one pancreatin tablet following each meal.
- Take one Alka-Aid antacid tablet 30 to 35 minutes after taking the pancreatin; take two tablets after a large meal.

The pancreatin tablet for aiding digestion contains 2400 mg pancreatin USP which provides the following enzyme activity:

- lipase (fat digesting) 12,000 USP units
- protease (protean digesting) 60,000 USP units
- amylase (starch digesting) 60,000 USP units

The Alka-Aid antacid lowers the hyperacidity and is made up of:

- sodium bicarbonate 360 mg
- potassium bicarbonate 180 mg

The follow-up instructions to this therapy said to:

"*CALL* this office in two weeks to let us know how you are progressing. Remind our staff member to enter your progress on your personal medical chart. Your progress is very important to both of us.

CONTINUE the same therapy unless adjustments are ordered by the doctor. If significant improvement has not occurred after three weeks, the doctor will review your chart, write adjustment orders, and you should report by telephone in seven days.

SIX MONTHS after you begin therapy, call (if you wish) for a repeat GASTROGRAM. Discontinue your therapy for seven days prior to coming in for this test."

The therapy resulting from the gastrogram test is doing well. The bloating after eating, belching, flatulence and gasiness in general has nearly vanished. Furthermore, I feel stronger, I can do more push-ups, so I must be benefiting from the absorption of more nutrients.

An interesting symptom typical of hyperacidity and slow emptying stomach is a constant feeling of hunger. That describes me perfectly before starting this therapy. As a result of this new regimen thus far my hunger is usually satisfied with three meals a day. My inclination to continually snack has diminished greatly.

As of this writing, I feel much better, but it has only been a short time.

The testing process starts with swallowing a small transmitter about the size of a large pill. The signal is picked up by an antenna placed on the stomach which makes the antenna resemble an oversized cummerbund. The signal transmits the amount of acidity which is then recorded on a time-graph.

The gastrogram approach is a significant improvement. The old method required stuffing a small tube down the throat into the stomach to extract some fluids for analysis. The tube routine could not extract fluids from the small intestine, nor could it tell the transit time for emptying the stomach.

The gastrogram instructions for patient preparation are detailed below:

Do not *eat* anything for 10 hours.

Do not *drink* anything for 10 hours.

If you eat or drink anything, it will render the test invalid. If you forgot and accidentally ate or drank something, call our office and tell our receptionist so you may be rescheduled.

When you arrive at the office, let our receptionist know you have been scheduled for a gastrogram.

When we know that you have arrived, we will then calibrate our gastrograph machine. This will take fifteen to twenty minutes.

The test is simple. You will be asked to swallow a capsule with a little water. *This is all you have to do.*

The capsule takes only a few seconds to reach your stomach. The pH (or amount of hydrochloric acid) of your stomach is automatically recorded.

The emptying time of people's stomachs varies from a few seconds to several hours. We have no way of knowing other than to do this test. However, whether your stomach empties fast or sluggishly, it is **important for the doctor to know.**

When the capsule empties into the small intestine, we will receive some very important pH data from you on our machine. Your reading should be in the neutral to alkaline range (non-acid). Vital digestive processes, including nutrient absorption, takes place in a *non-acid* medium.

Plan to spend from two to six hours. Bring something to keep you busy, like reading or knitting materials.

Remember . . . do not eat or drink anything for at least 10 hours!!

Heidelberg International, Norcross, Ga. are the distributors of the gastrogram machine.

CHAPTER 13

Odds & Ends

This is truly the odds and ends department. In my search for wellness, I came across a number of things of interest. What follows is a discussion on the subjects listed below:

- Lemon water—a simple but magical potion for better health
- Thermography—a diagnostic tool for doctors which will help them more accurately size up the problem and measure the progress of the treatment
- Homogenized Milk and Heart Disease. This theory relates to small molecules of fat absorbed by the intestine into the circulatory system which cause damage to the blood veins.
- Tongue scraping—This helps fight "dragon breath."
- Yeast Infection—otherwise known as candida albacans. A difficult problem to diagnose and treat.
- Reflexology—a country cousin to acupuncture or acupressure; a pleasurable experience

LEMON WATER

A small pamphlet entitled *Get the Big Picture About Health* distributed by Dr. John H. Gerath, tells about "lemon water."

When he says lemon, he means fresh lemon: not frozen, not Realemon, and not other citrus fruit such as lime.

The pamphlet says the juice from a fresh lemon diluted in eight ounces of distilled water has atomic power. It is a special form of vitamin C. Lemons regenerate the liver, strengthen stomach acids and salivary enzymes, and help the pancreas, thyroid and adrenal glands as well as other glands and organs of the body. It also strengthens the back because of the vitamin C.

The lemon juice must be diluted in water because the raw juice will eat the dentin off your teeth if there are any cracks in the enamel. Drink it one-half to one hour before eating. The average person should have one to three lemons per day. If the lemon water tastes sour it is indicative of high blood sugar levels. The author states continued use of the lemon water will return the blood sugar level to normal.

This pamphlet claims that lemon water is the most fantastic thing you can do to improve your health, increase your energy and prolong your life. If you take lemon water for the rest of your life you can add ten to thirty years to it. These are strong claims.

Albeit small, there is a perceptible improvement in the power of the stream when I pass water, I attribute this to the lemon water regimen.

By special permission from Dr. J. H. Gerath.

THERMOGRAPHY

The following description of thermography came from THERMA-SCAN, INC.

Medical Thermography is the science of obtaining and interpreting the information gained by a series of highly exact measurements of the skin's heat content in the form of a map. Medical Thermography is not a new science or process. Its value in the early detection of breast cancer and peripheral vascular and carotid artery insufficiencies was strongly indicated in 1956 and subsequently proven through the years by a team of dedicated physicians and engineers.

The living human body is a "heat generator" as a result of the inherent inefficiencies of normal metabolism. Most of this heat is generated in the viscera (internal organs) of the trunk where the processes of digestion and respiration as well as the action of the heart and liver occur. The more peripheral regions must derive the majority of their heat content from the viscera of the trunk which generates more heat than can be easily lost due to the smaller surface area/volume ratio. The means by which this heat flow is conducted from the viscera of the trunk to the peripheral regions such as the arms, legs, and head is the vascular system which reaches every living cell in the body.

The result of this heat flow from the viscera to the peripheral regions means that the blood of the arteries supplying the peripheral tissues will have a greater heat content than the blood of the veins draining the peripheral tissues. Further, vascular constriction and deficiencies to the peripheral regions can be quantitated by the reduced efficiency of the vas-

By special permission from Therma-Scan, Inc.

cular system as a distributor of heat. This means the areas behind or more peripheral to a constriction or blockage will have a reduced heat content (lower temperature) than normal range.

A cancer cell, because of its high growth rate and high metabolism, will have a higher heat content. If that cancer cell is in a breast or thyroid or any place not heavily insulated by the body wall, that heat content "floats" to the skin surface and can be detected as a warmer area. Further, cancer cells are usually found to inflame surrounding tissues as part of the body's immune response. Therefore, extremely small cancer growths can be detected by this site of inflammation coupled with the greater heat content of the venous system draining this area than the arterial system supplying it.

Arteriosclerosis is a disease which is usually systemic. This means no single artery or section of artery is afflicted by the clogging action of plaque—a hard mixture of calcium bound to cholesterol. This would indicate that the surgical replacement of an artery, as in a coronary bypass, would not solve the problem of insufficient vascular supply to the tissues. An artery is much like pipe as it does not directly supply any tissues, that takes place in a fine mesh of vessels called capillaries which are the site of supply to the tissues. Because of the small size and large surface area of the capillaries they are first to be obstructed by the deposition of plaque.

Every object in nature, however small or large, spontaneously radiates infrared energy as a function of its temperature. The warmer the object, the more intense is the infrared energy radiated.

By measuring the intensity of this radiation, one is able to determine the temperature of its source.

An infrared radiometer is a device with extreme accuracy. The Thermograph is a scanning infrared radiometer. As such, it is able not only to detect thousands of bits of temperature information per second, but it can display this information in the form of a "heat picture" or Thermogram.

The Thermogram is thus a quantitative and highly accurate composite expression of many thousands of separate temperature measurements.

It is not possible using conventional contact thermometers or thermocouples to measure precisely the temperature of an object at any given instant. This is true, because to touch an object is to disturb its thermal equilibrium and by definition, to change its temperature.

The Thermograph, on the other hand, is entirely passive. It measures temperature without contact—without influencing in any way the object under examination. For surface temperature measurement it is, therefore, the method par excellence.

Medical thermography is a source of information vital to the diagnosis and in the treatment of arteriosclerosis. Thus only medical thermography is able to provide a holistic dynamic monitor of the chelation therapy and determine the endpoint of treatment.

Thermography can help diagnose a wide variety of illnesses, and proves invaluable in monitoring developments in treatment and preventive processes.

Stroke. Thermography clearly shows the degree and location of the carotid obstruction before clinical symptoms occur. Post surgical monitoring of stroke victims is accomplished without the use of invasive dye injections, radiation, and anesthesia.

Pulmonary Embolism. Thermography diagnoses deep venous thrombosis in post operative patients prior to the appearance of clinical signs.

Orthopedics. Thermography is an early objective means to detect the soft tissue inflammation that invariable precedes tissue breakdown and ulceration. The regular monitoring of paraplegics, diabetics, and patients with insensitive limbs can prevent many amputations.

Burns. Thermography is an effective noncontact way of assessing the depth and scope of burns. It speeds surgical treatment and conclusively determines the viability of skin grafts.

Rheumatic Disease. Thermography indicates the extent of the inflammation and the effectiveness of therapy can be quantitatively measured by regular thermographic follow up of the patient without resorting to the use of invasive techniques.

Oncology. In addition to its contribution to the early detection of breast cancer, thermography is instrumental in localizing metastatic cancers and evaluation methods of therapy.

HOMOGENIZED MILK AND HEART DISEASE

Nicholas Sampsidis, M.S., author of a 32 page pamphlet titled *Homogenized,* Sunflower Publishing, Inc., makes a pretty convincing case. He points out that in 1900 heart disease in the U.S. was relatively rare. However, by 1950 heart disease became the number one killer.

He states cholesterol is taking a bum rap. He quotes Dr. Linus Pauling as saying, "I think this low cholesterol business is pretty much nonsense." Additionally a study of 1,700 patients (by Dr. Michael DeBakey, heart surgeon) who had atherosclerosis severe enough for hospitalization, only one patient in five had high serum cholesterol levels.

Mr. Sampsidis points out that an enzyme called xanthine oxidase (XO) is the principle culprit in an arterial occlusion. Some of the other ingredients are: triglycerides; phospholipids; and various minerals such as calcium; and the proteins, collagen and fibrin.

The XO is contained in milk fat. When milk is homogenized, the fat is broken up into very small particles, like mist in a fog. Some of the XO passes intact through the wall of the intestine and into the circulatory system. XO is an enzyme found in the liver where it is used to break down compounds like purine into uric acid. Humans have a natural storage of XO in the liver. However the XO from cow's milk that enters the blood stream creates havoc by attacking plasmalogen tissue within artery walls. Resulting from this attack are lesions within the artery wall and XO also attacks part of the heart muscle.

Your body responds to the XO-related damage by taking measures to protect the lesion from further attack. The scar tissue and calcified plaques represent the early stages of the healing process. The artery walls gradually thicken, obstructing the blood flow.

The progressive atherosclerosis process is started by XO from the homogenized milk. History shows that homogenized milk production began in 1932. Examination of Table 13–1 an extract from Table 1, page 11, from the pamphlet *Homoge-*

By special permission from Nicholas Sampsidis MS.

nized indicates an obvious correlation between milk intake, and percent homogenized, to the death rate from atherosclerosis. This presents a compelling argument.

The author is assisted by Dr. Kurt A. Oster in explaining this phenomenon. They present more proof of this from University of Delaware researchers.

HOMOGENIZED MILK HISTORY

	A	B	C
• Finland	244.7	593	90%
• United States	211.8	273	95%
• France	41.7	230	2%

A—Death rate per 100,000; B—Milk intake, pounds per person; C—approximate amount of homogenized milk.

Table 13-1

TONGUE SCRAPING

I learned this is an old Chinese hygiene routine. I tried this using a teaspoon as a scraper, amazed at the gunk that scraped off my tongue. I told a friend about this curiosity. He tried it because he had been bothered by "dragon breath" every morning. To his amazement, within about a week after adopting the habit of scraping his tongue morning and night, the dragon breath disappeared.

YEAST INFECTION

My dietitian, Bettina Esposito, former Chief Dietitian at The Center for Complementary Nutrition in New York City, enlightened me about the subject of yeast.

Your digestive tract serves as an environment for billions of good bacteria which help the digestive process and even manufacture some vitamins. In addition, lesser amounts of yeast and yet lesser quantities of "bad" bacteria, allergens, viruses, or parasites also call the digestive tract (and respiratory tract) "home." These latter organisms do not affect the healthy individual. However, should they increase in number disproportionately to the good bacteria, or if the immune system becomes weakened as the result of nutritional deficiencies, chemicals, molds, allergies, etc., health problems will occur.

Yeast, also called Candida Albicans, is especially able to multiply when certain antibiotics, steroids, or birth control pills are used. Their population growth results in the output of toxins which enter your bloodstream and further weaken the immune system. Until recently a diagnosis of "Candidiasis," the overabundance of yeast in your system, was somewhat subjective because health practitioners mostly depended upon symptoms presented more than laboratory results. Of course, my dietitian would not make a diagnosis because of her degree. However, after answering the long list of questions in a book by William Crook, M.D. called *The Yeast Connection*, GNC publication, this convinced me to change my diet. I asked Bettina for a list of foods which contain yeast or mold (because yeast can change into molds and vice versa) or may otherwise affect the growth of yeast in the digestive tract. You may be as surprised as I was to learn this includes many nutritious foods.

Many foods are believed to promote the growth of candida, and this is to be avoided. The list my dietitian gave me is indicated below.

- sugars of all kinds are at the head of the list; fructose

(fruit), sucrose, maltose, glucose, sorbitol, honey, molasses, maple and corn syrup
- yeast risen baked goods including bread, rolls, crackers, pita, pizza, etc.
- pickled vegetables
- peanuts and peanut butter; (fresh peanut butter should be OK)
- processed meats—luncheon meats, ham, bacon, sausage, etc.
- dairy products—cheese, sour cream, ice cream, etc. (milk in moderation—OK)
- condiments—ketchup, steak sauce, soy sauce, vinegar, malt, mayonnaise
- instant and regular coffee, tea and soft drinks
- refined flour products—breads and cakes
- enriched oatmeal—mostly baby foods

The above list is really bad news for food lovers. But for some, the worst is that alcoholic beverages of all kinds should be avoided.

The foods I could eat include:

- fresh fish, poultry, shellfish and eggs
- fresh vegetables, raw, or lightly steamed
- whole grains, non-yeast crackers or bread
- pumpkin and sunflower seeds/unhulled fresh nuts and seeds
- cold pressed oils; linseed, olive, safflower, sunflower, canola
- fresh fruits added cautiously to your diet low in cholesterol like melon, berries, grapefruit

My dietitian suggested the addition of a multiple vitamin, mineral, extra calcium/magnesium, and vitamin C to "fill in the gaps" created by my limited diet.

When symptom-free, the imbalance of the good and bad bacteria can be helped by taking acidophilus. Also, there are some things that can be taken to retard the yeast outgrowth. *YEASTOP* is one such item. A trip to your health food store may reveal other products that may be useful. However this is not a quick fix. Adjusting my diet and taking supplements is a slow process of turning things around.

REFLEXOLOGY

Reflexology is a form of acupressure. The left hand or foot pressure points mirror those of the right hand or foot. Putting fingertip pressure on the left and right foot stimulates whatever is connected. If the pressure point is painful, this could mean there is an imbalance or dysfunction of whatever point is under pressure. Some doctors use this technique as a diagnostic aid for small children. If you have no pain, supposedly you are reasonably healthy. A reflexologist usually will massage your feet for about 45 minutes. The theory is massaging the nerves stimulate the connecting glands and organs into better health. A 45 minute visit with a reflexologist working on your feet is a relaxing and soothing experience. Your health food store may offer a small plastic card identifying the location of nerves in your feet and hands that have connections to other parts of the body, such as, the heart, liver, lungs, sinus, eyes, brain, and so on.

CHAPTER 14

Hippocrates Health Institute

In the one year gap from the last chapter to this, my health profile deteriorated somewhat. It may have been because I backslid on my diet. Specifically, I started eating bread, pastry deserts (white flour and sugar); and used granola for breakfast on a regular basis. My weight edged up from 165 to 173 pounds.

Some of the old complaints reappeared, along with some new ones:

- The dry mouth, dry throat malady continued to be tolerable; except for brief periods.
- Nocturnal leg and foot cramps reappeared.
- The need to take pancreatic enzyme tablets to aid in the digestive process continued. If I forgot to take them after eating, indigestion soon followed.
- I developed a daily recurring pain in my abdomen and it remained undiagnosed for about eight months prior to my experience at Hippocratic Health Institute.

- I quickly got nauseated every time I tried to exercise flat on my back.
- My cholesterol climbed to 238, even though I was on a low fat diet.
- I suffered from a stiff neck for about ten months in spite of chiropractic treatments.

THE SEARCH GOES ON:

The search led me to the Hippocrates Health Institute (HHI), West Palm Beach, Florida. I enrolled in their three week guest program (Dec. 17, 1988 to Jan. 7, 1989) over the Christmas and New Year holiday season. I learned of many things that contribute to the achievement of wellness.

The diverse make-up of the guest list included:

- 27 year old young man from South Africa
- 22 year old young woman from London
- 74 year old couple from Switzerland
- 70 year old woman from Germany
- 28–30 year old couple with 3 children from Minnesota
- 60 year old woman from California
- 63 year old woman from Florida
- 70–73 year old couple from Maryland
- 74 year old man from Virginia
- 66 year old man from Virginia; Kansas Mattson (the ages noted above are my best guess)

We soon felt like one big family as we got to know each other. Five of the guests had previously gone through this program and were back for a refresher.

Monday through Friday we kept busy from about 6 a.m. to 10:30 p.m. A typical day followed this schedule—

6:00 a.m.	enema and wheatgrass juice implant
8:00 a.m.	exercise
9:00 a.m.	breakfast
9:30 a.m.	classes
11:45 a.m.	lunch
1:00 p.m.	classes
4:30 p.m.	free time
5:30 p.m.	dinner
7:00 p.m.	special guest lectures
9:00 p.m.	enema and wheatgrass implant
10:30 p.m.	retire

The many facets of the Hippocrates program are under the guidance of Brian R. Clement, Director. The regimen is aimed at cleansing and detoxifying your body. The different subjects/activities I will discuss are noted below. The colon cleansing program is an important part of the Hippocrates Health encounter which I will address as a separate subject in the next chapter.

- Living Food diet and juice fasting
- Wheatgrass juice detoxification
- Daily exercise classes
- Medical testing monitored by Jack Schocoff, M.D., a medical consultant
- The body's elimination systems
- Chiropractic treatments
- Massage therapy
- Food combining/food preparation classes
- Why vegetarianism?
- Mental health
- Recreational outings

THE LIVING FOOD DIET

The cornerstone of the Hippocrates Health program is the living food diet. Living food means eating everything uncooked. The reason for this is because cooking with a temperature above 115°F. kills the enzymes in the food. This is called "dead food" by the Institute which says that such food is less nutritious and harder to digest. Previous research has also shown processing and cooking significantly depletes the vitamin content of food.

The diet includes a list of no-no's, no:

—white flour
—sugar
—salt
—caffeine
—meat, animal, fowl or fish
—peanuts or peanut butter
—dairy (milk, butter and cheese products)
—chocolate
—alcohol
—tobacco

Buckwheat and pumpkin seed sprouts together with fresh vegetables are the staples of the diet. Dulse, a seaweed, is used as a supplement. It contains important trace minerals, iodine and iron.

In between meals "green drinks" made from buckwheat and pumpkin seed sprouts and an assortment of vegetables (carrots, celery, cucumber, turnip, beets, zucchini) are used as a snack. The green drinks are loaded with vitamins and minerals that are readily absorbed into the body.

Other fundamentals observed by the Hippocrates diet are:

- Breakfast is fresh fruit juice, or occasionally fresh fruit. The body is still in its cleansing cycle, and the fruit helps this process.

- Juice fasting once a week to give your body a rest and give it a chance to cleanse itself.

To summarize, the living food diet includes these basic elements.

+ The list of no-no's
+ Living food (raw fruit, vegetables and nuts)
+ Two eight ounce green drinks a day from fresh sprouts and vegetables
+ Juice fasting one day per week
+ Daily exercise

WHEATGRASS JUICE DETOXIFICATION

Wheatgrass is sprouted wheat. When five or six days old, it reaches a height of about six inches. This is cut and processed by a special machine to make the juice.

Wheatgrass juice promotes the detoxification process. It is a rich source of vitamin A, B and C. It is 70% chlorophyll and contains the essential amino acids the body needs. Wheatgrass juice is also rich in calcium, iron, sulphur, cobalt, potassium, sodium and zinc.

The chlorophyll content of wheat grass juice is similar to hemoglobin. The difference is the blood contains the iron as a metallic atom, whereas chlorophyll contains magnesium. Chlorophyll is given credit for the following goodness:

- Arrests growth and development of unfriendly bacteria
- Aids in rebuilding the bloodstream
- Inhibits the metabolic activation of carcinogens
- Normalizes blood sugar levels
- Promotes tissue cell activity and its normal regrowth

- Increases production of hemoglobin
- Helps counteract ingested toxins

The wheatgrass juice with its vitamins, mineral and chlorophyll content has a triple nutrient value. Wheatgrass juice has been found to be effective for a number of conditions as indicated below. However, to realize these powerful results it is recommended to be consumed within twenty minutes of extracting the juice.

- Excess amounts of toxic metals can be lowered (lead, cadmium, mercury, aluminum and copper)
- Neutralize guanidine, a toxic chemical released through trauma
- Wheatgrass juice poultices are good for sores and boils, cuts, burns and insect bites
- Drinking it reduces high blood pressure
- Using it as an *implant* accelerates the detoxification process; it cleanses and heals the internal organs

DAILY EXERCISE

Five days a week, one hour each day. Four of the five days, aerobic exercise, and one day yoga exercise. Alix Weill, a vivacious woman in her mid-sixties, the exercise instructor/cheerleader, says flexible muscles are young muscles. Alix presented a good example for us to emulate.

During the last fifteen to twenty minutes of some of the exercise classes, Alix gave instructions on ballroom dancing. Besides being fun, it was good exercise.

We had one exercise class in the swimming pool. The resistance the water presents serves to tone muscle and increase strength.

I learned one of the important reasons why you need to exercise. The flexing of the muscles pulses the lymph nodes and glands which aids the lymphatic system in eliminating toxic body waste. Exercise is essential to the body's basic metabolism. Now I am more motivated to exercise everyday.

The Hippocrates Health Institute recommends the use of a small trampoline (rebounder) twenty minutes per day. This is reported to be an excellent method to exercise the lymphatic system. I bought one as soon as I got home from Hippocrates. I worked this into my routine doing it just before going to bed. As a result, my sleep seems to be more restful. I also use it after meals. Somewhat like "burping the baby." It gets rid of the air I swallowed during eating.

MEDICAL TESTING

On the second day after our arrival and the second from the last day before departure we had extensive blood tests done. Blood pressure readings and our weight were recorded once a week. A private consultation with the doctor afforded the opportunity to discuss personal health issues.

My significant "before" and "after" readings were:

	BEFORE	AFTER
Weight	173	159
Cholesterol	222	173
Blood pressure	90/60	100/70
	Borderline anemic	Borderline anemic
Blood sugar	low	low

The weight loss is kind of curious, I lost one pound per day for the first ten days then tapered off to 1/2 pound a day.

Heretofore with diets, I lost up to five or six pounds the first two days then leveled off. The decrease in the cholesterol is typical of those who partake in the living food diet. Blood pressure is in a good range, but my borderline anemia and low blood sugar will take more than three weeks to turn around. After all, it took more than three weeks to get into this condition.

THE BODY'S ELIMINATION SYSTEMS

Our body's chemical factory is meant to be self-cleaning and self-healing. However, I tended to put various parts of the system to a handicap during my lifetime. The Hippocrates program reminded me that the body has these elimination systems:

- The colon is the main channel for eliminating digested foods, dead tissue cells, living and dead bacteria. (Colon health is further discussed in Chapter 15.)
- The blood is circulated through the liver and lungs to eliminate the toxic materials.
- The other body fluids are filtered by the kidneys and eliminated through the bladder. The health of the reproductive organs can affect the functioning of the urinary tract.
- I know that the skin is an organ, but I seem to forget it needs daily attention. Hippocrates recommends dry brushing the skin to promote the elimination of dead skin and, at the same time, help to stimulate the lymphatic system.
- I also knew there is a lymphatic system. What I did not know is that the lymphatic system does not have a pump such as the heart for the circulatory system. Physical movement is necessary to activate it. The diaphragm is sometimes called the lymphatic pump, so we had breathing exercises to learn how to take advantage of this. Addi-

tionally, exercise such as walking, bicycling, rebounding, and swimming increase the lymph flow to nourish the body and eliminate toxins. It finally struck home, exercise is necessary to keep the lymphatic system functioning for good health. Conversely, lack of exercise delays the removal of toxic waste and impedes the distribution of nutrients to the body.

CHIROPRACTIC TREATMENTS

Dr. Bob, the chiropractor, made treatments available to those who felt they had the need. I had three treatments for my stiff neck. A perceptible improvement resulted with each treatment. However, the results were short-lived; typically about 24 hours. It seemed like five steps forward and three steps back. The cumulative effects resulted in relieving about 25% of the stiffness. I think it is fair to say that continued improvement could be expected if I could have stayed on for more treatments.

Dr. Bob had an interesting approach in his treatment protocol. He started with a reflexology examination of the feet to get a picture of the individual's general health. His examination also revealed I had a clogged up transverse colon after the masseuse identified the same condition earlier unbeknownst to him—see Chapter 15.

MASSAGE THERAPY

Norma Vega, a native of Mexico, the licensed massage therapist, was a most delightful person. She changed her occupation from a certified public accountant (CPA) to a masseuse because it was more profitable and more enjoyable.

There are several different techniques employed in body massage. Her technique included applied reflexology.

The full body massage went on for sixty minutes. Besides relaxing, and loosening tight muscles, the process also stimulated the lymphatic system's elimination of toxins.

The tuition included one massage per week, and extras were made available at added cost. Everybody, went for the extras, and so Norma worked a full appointment calendar.

FOOD COMBINING/FOOD PREPARATION CLASS

We had classroom lectures on food combining and again in the kitchen during the food preparation classes.

The food combining ground rules are discussed below. The food preparation details are presented in Appendix C with various recipes.

Food combining got my attention because of the problems with my digestive system. In particular, my pancreas was not functioning up to par. When I failed to follow the food combining ground rules, even with taking enzyme tablets, my digestive system got upset.

Food combining is based on the principle that different classes of food require a combination of different enzymes, acids and times to be digested.

Some of the basic rules of food combining break with traditional American eating habits.

- Fruits, in general, should be eaten on an empty stomach.

- Proteins and starches generally do not combine well, an example is steaks and baked potatoes.
- Proteins and starches, individually mix well with vegetables.
- Fruits are classed as acid, sub-acid and sweet. Combining fruits is classed as fair. Acid and sub-acid fruits take 1 to 1 1/2 hours to digest while sweet fruit takes three to four hours.
- Sweet fruit and starches are a poor mix. Now consider the traditional fruitcake with protein (nuts), starches (flour), and fruit, a double poor mix. When I eat a fruitcake now I know why it feels "heavy on the stomach."

There is an abundance of information on this subject available in most health food stores, including detailed charts and books.

WHY VEGETARIANISM?

Hippocrates' regimen is classed as a "Living Food Vegetarian Diet." The definition is: "One who eats only raw vegetables, fruit, nuts, seeds and grains, with particular emphasis on sprouted seeds and grains, as well as fermented enzyme rich foods such as seed cheeses and sauerkraut.

Hippocrates Institute pointed out some of the reasons for vegetariansim. This comparison is most interesting and convincing. Generally, studies have shown vegetarians are healthier than meat eaters:

Health Reasons

- Vegetarian athletes can engage in more vigorous activity two to three times longer than meat eaters

- During World War II many countries experienced meat shortages, and people were forced to adopt a mainly vegetarian diet. The death rate dropped dramatically, coupled with a marked decrease in disease.
- In the Journal of the American Medical Association of June 3, 1961, an article on heart disease, made this statement, "A vegetarian diet can prevent 90% of thrombo embolic disease [clot obstruction in veins] and 97% of coronary occlusions [closed up veins and arteries]."
- Studies among 7th Day Adventists and Mormons who are mainly vegetarians show them to have half as many incidences of degenerative diseases as the rest of the population.

Physiological Comparisons

All indications point to the human body's being created to assimilate vegetation rather than meat.

TEETH: Carnivores have fangs and teeth especially suitable for tearing off chunks of meat. Their jaws move only up and down, without any side to side grinding capability. Herbivores (that's us) have flat back molars for grinding food and jaws that move both up and down and sideways permitting more thorough mastication.

DIGESTIVE TRACT: The entire digestive tract in a human is from 32 to 36 feet long, starting at the mouth and ending at the rectum. A straight line from the mouth to the rectum might measure from $2^1/_2$ to 3 feet in the average adult. It means that food travels ten to twelve times that distance during the digestive process. In *meat-eating animals,* the digestive system measures only one and a half times the distance from the mouth to the rectum. Carnivores digest their food much more quickly, eliminating waste products before putrefaction can take place. They secrete more hydrochloric acid to break down the meat into amino acids. The food eaten by humans remains in the body six times longer, so meat-eating humans create bodily imbalances by forcing the digestive system to produce abnormal amounts of hydrochloric acid. This causes over-acidity throughout the entire digestive tract bringing on physical difficulties.

SMALL INTESTINE COMPARISON: The inside walls of the small intestines of meat-eating animals are fairly smooth and are quite short, allowing food to pass through quickly. The length of the small intestine in the average human is about twenty-two feet and is about one inch in diameter. Inside there are thousands of little fingers called villi. As the food travels through the small intestine, the nutrients filter down between the villi and are absorbed into the bloodstream. Dairy products and dense proteins, like meat, generate great amounts of mucus in the stomach and small intestines interfering with the absorption of nutrients. The pockets in the colon also become coated with this sludge leaving less and less room for the food to pass through. Eating lots of spicy food irritates the membranes and causes even more mucus to be secreted to protect the intestinal walls from these irritants. All this mucus seriously impedes the absorption of nutrients, and the body progressively becomes starved, aging rapidly and resulting in a weakened immune system. By eliminating mucus-forming dairy, eggs, and meat, and adopting a vegetarian diet, the body gradually cleanses itself and is better able to absorb more and more nutrients from the food.

MENTAL HEALTH

Timothy O'Higgins, psychologist from Ireland, who was a visiting member of the Hippocrates Health Institute staff, gave one of the evening programs.

Timothy made a lot of sense on life and living. The highlights from his talk are noted below. I find these powerful statements and something to think about.

- Whatever we judge, we perpetuate.
- When emotion is attached to thought, the reaction multiplies.
- Emotion is regenerative or degenerative.
- Use it or lose it:
  +the mind as a healer
  +the mind as a medicine—miracles happen
- Why hold onto what is not yours, unhook; forgiveness works wonders.
- Anger is good, but do not become an angry person.
- The first stage of healing is recognition.
- Let go of that internal judgment.
- Whatever you give your mind to, it has you.

In another class on mental health, I gleaned the following statements—more food for thought.

- Growth is a process of experimentation
- You will know you have learned a lesson when your actions change
- If you are alive, there are lessons to be learned (almost everyday)
- Take charge of your life or someone else will

RECREATIONAL OUTINGS

It was not all work and no play. Mid-week, Saturdays and Sundays, were times for special outings. We visited two of the beaches on three different occasions. We spent one evening in downtown West Palm Beach at a place for dancing.

On another evening, we went to the Enquirer Corporation Headquarters to view one of the largest Christmas lighting displays in the world. They claimed their Christmas tree to be the tallest in the U.S. The extravaganza and beauty of it all presented a fairyland to behold. It attracted thousands.

On Christmas Day, the Hippocrates staff went all out in putting on a Christmas banquet. Many of us had visits from friends and relatives. My son and his wife, together with their five children, participated in this event, a joyous occasion.

The Hippocrates staff also held a special program for New Year's Eve.

All of these events helped to nourish the spirit to keep things in balance with the activities that worked on the physical health.

MY PERSONAL ASSESSMENT

The Hippocrates Health Institute has a well-balanced, interesting program. The staff answered questions and helped as needed. They give meaning to the slogan, "We Care"; they really do!

The diet and exercise, coupled with the concern for colon health, has to be the fastest way to purge yourself of toxins. The diagnosis of the pain in my abdomen and getting on the path to restoring my colon to a healthy state relieved some anxiety. It delighted me to rapidly come down to the "desired" weight for my height—and stay there with no problems; and to see my cholesterol drop forty-nine points.

I would not hesitate to recommend this program to anybody in search of improving his health.

CHAPTER 15

Colon Health

Colon health may be an ignoble subject for polite dinner conversation. It is one of the best kept secrets in this country, but this should not be the case.

Hippocrates Health Institute places great emphasis on colon cleansing as a part of the detoxification process. I have some memories and experience relating to colon health problems.

- My son, at age 46, got a severe case of colitis that his doctors were unable to cure except by surgical intervention. He now wears a bag as a result of the ileostomy. I lived, and am living with him in this experience, so I have some appreciation and insight into this kind of situation.
- Two close friends lost a major section from their colon because of malignancy. One caught it in time; the other friend was too late, his cancer had fully metastisized.
- Two other friends had little more than a straight pipe left after their doctors used surgical intervention to resolve severe cases of diverticulitis.

Fortunately, my colon problems were less severe. I suffered through diverticulitis episodes in earlier years, but learned how to keep it under control. I gained a better understanding of the need for colon health from the following analysis. This discovery at age 65 is certainly too soon old, too late smart.

SYMPTOMS

- An eight-month history of pain across my abdomen, laterally, about two inches above the navel; not my stomach, it was something else. The dull pain came and went at various times during the day; day after day. I adjusted my diet some five years ago and since that time I have not suffered from constipation. Nor was I able to make any association of the pain with my diet or when I ate.
- I suffered sharp pains in my lower right groin I believed to be my prostate (I could be confusing this with the appendix). These would come and go but happened often enough to be disquieting. The high incidence of prostate cancer kept me coming back on a regular basis for a checkup.
- I had a history of rapidly becoming nauseated when trying to do physical exercise when lying flat on my back; like situps or leg lifts. This had no apparent linkage to the pain in my abdomen; I would get nauseated whether or not I had any pain.
- I also had a stiff neck. This resulted in considerable immobility and sore muscles.

DIAGNOSIS

The above four complaints were presented to my family doctor for his assessment.

- Family Doctor (M.D.)—prostate checked normal. Examination of the abdomen revealed no abnormalities. After a discussion of my pains and lifestyle, the doctor gave me the impression that my problems were stress-related. Remove the stress and the pains will go away, but I did not buy this theory.
- Hippocrates Health Institute—about two weeks later:
  + Masseuse—during a full body massage diagnosed my pain as a clogged up colon. I said, "You're kidding, I have no problems with bowel movements!" "I am a regular guy." She proceeded to mark out the area with her fingers. To my amazement, she precisely outlined the area of the pain across my abdomen that I complained about. Then, she went to the inside of the heel on my right foot and rapidly confirmed her diagnosis from a reflexology pressure point. "You need five or six colonics to get cleaned out," she told me. (It took five. In reality, you keep taking colonics until you come clean.)
  + Hippocrates Health Institute chiropractor. Dr. Bob used reflexology to get an idea of the patient's health before making an adjustment. He rapidly identified the transverse colon as a problem.
  + Colonic therapist at West Palm Beach also used the reflexology technique to understand the health of the colon. The ascending and descending checked normal, but the reflexology pressure point confirmed the diagnosis of the clogged transverse colon.

TREATMENT

At the Hippocrates Health Institute three week health renewal program, we accomplished high enemas first thing in the morning and the last thing at night using a twenty-two inch probe. A wheatgrass juice implant (four ounces of fresh wheatgrass juice, undiluted, implanted in the colon using the same apparatus as used for the enema) followed each enema. I completed about twenty-five of these treatments that yielded a lot of mucus and flaking of particles, but the diagnosis revealed the transverse colon still needed help.

The colonic therapist inserted a disposable plastic speculum into the anus two to three inches. This fixture included an inlet pipe to let gravity-fed water flow in. The other part was an exhaust pipe to allow evacuation of the colon by suction. The water cycled in and out through a clear plastic pipe to allow the monitoring of the waste products.

- The first treatment resulted in more mucus and mostly small flaky fecal matter.
- The second treatment removed large black chunks of debris that appeared to come from the folds in the colon. As the water cycled in and out, the therapist either massaged or used a mechanical vibrator over the colon to help dislodge the residue.

BACK HOME

Two were done in West Palm Beach, but I needed two or three more to complete the program. The search for colonic therapy began with the Yellow Pages. I found none listed in a metropolitan area of 400,000 people. A call to a large hospital doctors' referral service yielded, "We don't list colonics in our service directory." I am told that years ago enemas were a familiar treatment of the old fashioned country doctor; but enemas are now disdained by modern physicians who gravitate toward the use of high-tech equipment.

After more searching, as if these people were part of an underground, I found two places.

PREPARATION FOR COLONICS AND AFTER CARE

I realized after I returned home the Hippocrates Health Institute routine of twice daily enemas keeps the colon empty and ready for colon irrigation. Starting with an empty colon helps the process. The following are suggestions by my second colonic therapist.

- A series of abdominal castor oil packs, one each day for one hour, for the three days preceding the colonic. Also, a teaspoon of olive oil in a cup of hot water for three nights at bedtime. The castor oil pack is a soft cotton cloth, like a diaper, impregnated with castor oil. This is spread over the abdomen with a heating pad on top. I placed a pillow on top of this to hold in the heat. Caution is needed as it is possible to get the heat too high causing minor burns.
- Take a laxative the day before the colonic; or
- An enema the night before. An increased diet of naturally laxative foods several days before the colonic helps. Some examples include fresh, raw fruits and vegetables, bran, and dried fruits.
- Do not eat one and a half hours prior to the colonic as it may make the colonic uncomfortable. Note—for those on a special diet or taking medication at mealtime, disregard the instructions on not eating.

I used castor oil packs and a series of enemas the morning of the colonic, which worked well. I could see this with the enemas and the colonics that followed. An uncommon amount of mucus discharge came from treatments four and five.

POST COLONIC TREATMENT

The post-colonic therapy suggestions are made from four different aspects: 1) to keep you comfortable; 2) to replenish the good bacteria (flora); 3) to restore the electrolytes; and 4) other—

The "keep you comfortable" suggestions include:

- avoid strenuous exercise the day of the colonic
- avoid alcohol, and gas-producing foods such as beans and cabbage; and
- have a light meal.

To replenish the flora, yogurt and buttermilk are recommended. Also acidophilus milk or acidophilus capsules are helpful in this regard.

The restoration of the elecytrolyte is realized by intake of fresh fruits and vegetables or juices. Also foods high in calcium and potassium are helpful.

Another suggestion is to take "Perfect 7" for three days following a colonic. This will clean out residual mucus and other debris and aid in the healing process. Perfect 7 is a powdered mixture including psyllium seed, rose hips, buckthorn bark, golden seal and capsicum. It seems to work and it is highly recommended by the colonic therapist and Hippocrates Health Institute. Perfect 7 is available in most health food stores.

My colonic therapist advised that a dirty colon does not work too well, and whether or not it will lose all of its flora and electrolytes from the colonic treatment is of no great concern. The urgent matter is to get the colon clean so it can be restored to health. From their experiences, both therapists explained the "threat of losing the flora and electrolytes" is a scare tactic that does not hold up in actual practice. The post-colonic instructions are added insurance.

To maintain colon health, HHI recommends:

- weekly enemas
- avoidance of mucus producing foods (discussed earlier); and
- alternate the use of Perfect 7, three days on followed by three days off; every other month.

OBSERVATIONS ON COLON HEALTH

- The pain across the abdomen, the pain I thought to be the prostate, and nausea I experienced in the past disappeared within two days of completing the five colonic series.
- The perpetual "tired look" that my friends constantly reminded me of is gone.
- I seem to have more energy, a spring in my step.
- Dr. Norman Walker, author of *Colon Health* wrote a convincing book which I ordered to send to my family and friends. A fellow Hippocrates Health Institute attendee who thought the same as I, did likewise. "I'm not constipated so what's the problem?" he told me. He promptly signed up for colonics after reading the book. He also bought ten copies to send to his family and friends. (Dr. Walker reportedly lived to be more than one hundred years old, and did not die from natural causes, but from injuries sustained in an accident.)
- Among other things, Dr. Walker illustrates how the colon is connected to all the other parts of the body: e.g. organs, eyes, ears, glands, etc. The fluid from the colon is absorbed in the body through the colon wall by osmosis. A colon impacted with fecal matter will also transmit toxins during the osmosis process. Then these toxins have to be accommodated by the liver and kidneys or lymphatic sys-

tem as they process the body fluids or the body gets overloaded with toxins. As I see it, it is difficult to become healthy and to stay healthy with an impacted colon. I wondered how much longer my body could have stood this insult before disease set in.

- "Why?"
  + Why don't the M.D.'s pay attention to colon health to avoid the need for crisis treatment?
  + Why aren't they more attuned to diagnosis by touch (similar technique to their examination of the liver); and by reflexology pressure points?
  + Why isn't the public better informed on this subject?

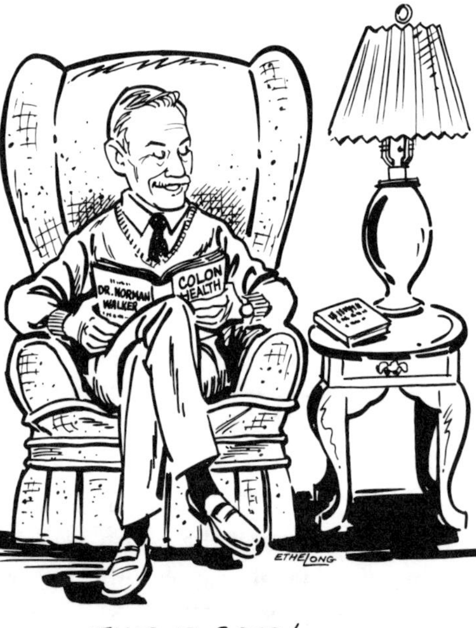

THIS IS GOOD!

- I am convinced colon health should be treated in a preventive maintenance sense. I can't help but believe my long history of malabsorption may have a direct relationship to my colon problem. Only time will tell if this thesis is correct. I wonder if I would have had diverticulitis, or if my son and friends would have had their difficulties if we all had been attuned to the need for colon health maintenance.

If you are interested in pursuing this matter, try the Yellow Pages under "colonics". If that does not work, call 1-800-237-8458, POTOLO Research, if you want to find someone who offers colon irrigation services in your area.

CHAPTER 16

Dry Mouth Cure

It seems as though prophetic justice is being served—I started the book with a dry mouth problem, and end with a cure.

As stated earlier, my original dry mouth condition realized substantial improvement from vitamin supplementation. However, at sporadic intervals I continued to suffer, although the frequency and severity did not match the original complaint. So the search went on for a more complete cure. Note, when I say dry mouth, that includes the throat; a dryness in the throat makes it difficult to talk or swallow.

Quite unexpectedly, I got a telephone call from Pauline, my chelation nurse. She excitedly relayed the experience of her husband. She described his condition as being severe, having to wash his food down with water otherwise he could not swallow. Pauline said that in less than five minutes the doctor had her husband salivating so profusely that he had to lean over a sink. But Mean Pauline, true to her name, would not tell me how the doctor made this happen. She said find out for yourself. Dr. William Root, a dentist in Charlottesville, Virginia has the answer.

So I called the next day. It pleased me to hear the receptionist say Dr. Root did indeed know how to cure dry mouth problems.

Dr. Root found most of the dry mouth conditions can be traced to a person's "bite." An adjustment in the bite normally corrects this situation. The bite adjustment is done with the aid of an orthodonic appliance fitted in the rear of the bite.

So on my first visit with Dr. Root, he quickly demonstrated his technique. He placed two wads of dental wax both sides at the rear of my mouth. Then he instructed me to bite down a little and hold it. At the time, my mouth and throat were somewhat dry, but to my astonishment, the saliva began to flow and my mouth *and* throat instantly became moist.

Dr. Root then made impressions of my mouth to facilitate the fabrication of the orthodonic appliance. I returned in about three weeks to get fitted with the appliance. I am grateful to Dr. Root for correcting this troublesome condition. I hope that this dental procedure is being taught to dental students.

Dr. Root explained to me not only is a misaligned bite a causitive factor for dry mouth, it is also implicated in other dysfunctions. Although the jaw muscles are not directly linked to the back of the neck, he believes there are reflected forces that affect the top of the spine by muscle contractions and/or spasms when the bite is out of alignment. These contractions or spasms also can affect a major center of control of the sympathetic nervous system located near the base of the skull. When this occurs, what happens next is not always predictable. Dr. Root cited a number of cases to prove his point.

Case A. Dr. Root himself suffered from unexplained severe headaches until he made the discovery of his misaligned bite. He said now when he feels one of those headaches come on, he puts the orthodonic fixture in his mouth and the onset of the headache is stopped.

Case B. A lady from Arkansas who experienced a constant headache for ten years realized relief by using Dr. Root's technique.

Case C. A professional golfer experienced back pains that interfered with his game. Chiropractic adjustments did not help. Dr. Root reasoned that the reflected force caused a spinal misalignment. Dr. Root resolved the problem by adjusting this golfer's bite with an orthodonic appliance.

Case D. Described as a man with problems similar to mine, dry mouth and stiff neck. Although the dry mouth problem quickly resolved itself, the stiff neck condition lingered on. In the sixth month, Case D experienced a "popping" in the neck and the pains immediately dissipated. So maybe there is some hope for my stiff neck. (My misalignment is between C-1 and C-2, the top two vertabrae in my neck.)

In addition to the cases cited above, Dr. Root's technique of correcting the bite works as a cure for tic douloureux (trigeminal neuralgia). This is a searing pain that comes to the side of the face. The pain may last from one to fifteen minutes or longer. These attacks happen at random times and frequency.

It may go into remission for a period, then return with lightning jabs of pain. Dr. Root said his success rate for treating this malady is 85 to 90%.

Although my experience with the orthodonic appliance is limited, I feel like I am cured. It is a pleasure to have a moist mouth and throat. Besides that, the orthodonic appliance makes a good conversation piece.

Dr. Root welcomes any inquiry. He can be contacted at:

Charlottesville, VA
(804) 293–5148

CHAPTER 17

So What Have I Learned

In my search for wellness I have learned the aging process and personal health can be controlled. It takes self-discipline and an earnest desire to become knowledgeable about how to achieve and maintain a state of *wellness*. However, *one must take personal responsibility* for one's health and well-being; this cannot be delegated. The rewards are enormous. Once you have achieved a state of *wellness* you can accomplish more and realize greater enjoyment out of life.

What I have learned is presented from three different perspectives: (It is difficult to make such a presentation without some obvious redundancies.)

- causal factors for my problems
- cures
- other interesting health facts.

CAUSAL FACTORS

Significant causal factors impacting my health besides an improper diet include:

- the *food allergy* connection to arthritis, constipation and energy level
- *mercury amalgams* in my teeth, and how they stressed my neurological system
- lack of *exercise* and how it influenced weight control and energy level in a negative way.
- *malabsorption* of nutrients, and how subtle this is. This probably has been with me for years but went undiagnosed.
- *negative thoughts* like the ones below:
  + "Boy, am I tired!" This used to be repeated every morning as I sat on the edge of the bed, and several other times during the day.
  + "Gee, am I hungry!" I said about fifteen minutes every time after getting up from a good meal. (In fairness to myself, the malabsorption problem may have contributed to this.)
  + "The dysfunctions happening to me are a part of the normal aging process." (This is the *big lie* of our times.)

CURES

My health problems are recapitulated below together with what I experienced as the cure.

PROBLEM	CURE
• chronic constipation	food allergy diet and dietary bulk

• urinary tract disorder/ nightly bathroom trips	chiropractic treatment—spinal alignment, and lemon water
• sinus drainage	abstinence from milk
• weight control	food allergy diet and exercise
• cold hands/feet	vitamin supplements and chelation therapy
• prostatic enlargement	zinc supplement
• diverticulitis	abstinence from milk
• nocturnal leg/foot cramp	vitamin B-6 and calcium
• chronic fatigue	vitamin/mineral supplements and attitude change
• cold sores	vitamin and mineral supplements
• muscle spasms	calcium, magnesium, potassium
• dry nasal passages	vitamin/mineral supplements
• dry eyes	vitamin A
• hemorrhoids	elimination of constipation
• stomach ulcer	diet control
• brittle nails	zinc and calcium
• bursitis	uncertain
• arthritis	food allergy diet (elimination of beef)
• dry mouth	vitamin A, C, B complex
• flatulence	food allergy diet and bringing digestive pH into proper balance, control of candida
• hardening of arteries	chelation therapy and low fat diet
• malabsorption	food allergy diet; stomach and intestinal pH are part of the answer. The other elements are elusive, suspect proper vitamin and mineral balance
• short term memory and inability to concentrate	(1) Chelation therapy to eliminate toxic aluminum (2) Elimination of mercury amalgam

• weak lower leg muscles	chelation therapy to restore circulation
• xerosis	ditto above
• drift of resting pulse rate to an abnormally low reading	chelation therapy (but I don't know why)

OTHER INTERESTING HEALTH FACTS

The identification and/or expansion of the items listed below did not fit neatly into the two preceding topic headings. However, these items are of some importance.

Arthritis

I once thought that arthritis was hereditary because of my mother's problems with her hands. However, I found by diet it is possible to arrest the further spread of the soreness in the joints. By diet I have kept my arthritic joints pain-free without the need for painkillers.

I do not believe my experience is isolated. I know of other people who have achieved results similar to mine. My conviction that arthritis is avoidable or controllable through diet is reinforced by Dr. Marshall Mandell's book *5 Day Allergy Relief System.*

In my opinion, control of arthritis by diet is the best way. Controlling the pain by drugs does nothing to arrest the growth of arthritis. The drugs inevitably lead to side effects and results in further complicating one's health.

Food Allergies

Food allergies can cause a number of difficulties including:

- chronic fatigue
- sinus drainage
- obesity and food addiction
- arthritis
- skin problems
- insomnia
- difficulty with digestion
- confusion, depression, memory loss

Dr. Stuart Berger revealed his struggle with a severe case of obesity. As related earlier in Chapter 5, Berger overcame his weight problem after identifying the offending foods. Dr. Berger fortifies my own experience. Weight control has ceased to be a problem since I learned of my food allergies.

My digestive problems, specifically constipation, had a linkage to beef.

My continually draining sinuses were directly linked to milk. This problem was solved more than six years ago after I stopped drinking milk.

This list could go on and on. I have learned that food allergies, or perhaps more distinctly food intolerance, is the cause of many difficulties with one's health. Many times the body's reaction to the offending food is so subtle it goes unnoticed until there is an unpleasant manifestation such as colitis, diverticulitis, arthritis or some other problem. Allergy symptoms are not limited to runny eyes or nose, itching, or sneezing.

Resting Pulse Rate (RPR)—a function of diet and exercise

RPR is one of the common and accepted measures of one's health status. A RPR in the mid-60s is considered normal. Diet and exercise, or a lack thereof, can have a dramatic influence on the RPR. The object is to attain a lower reading through proper diet and exercise, thus resulting in lowering the number of heartbeats which means less stress on the heart, and a longer life.

A history of my RPR notes a decline in how hard my heart works; thirty percent less than it did before I started my program.

- about 65 RPR before starting the diet and exercise program.
- lower 50s RPR resulted from a faithful walking program.
- forty-two to 44 RPR within six months of starting my jogging program. My RPR frequently drifted as low as 36 as I sat in conferences, but I don't consider this as a healthy situation.

The RPR is an interesting thing if one pays attention to it. I can validate Coca's experience that the RPR is an accurate indicator of food intolerance. A rise of eight to ten beats per minute within fifteen minutes of eating a food is the signal. It usually rises within two or three minutes. This signal indicates a food intolerance, and indeed it makes your heart work harder. It does not necessarily give a clue as to how the reaction will manifest itself should you choose to continue eating food(s) to which you are allergic. This is why the food diary is important. By making notes on how you feel during the course of a day, it is possible to track down the food culprit.

When I get off my diet on a daily basis, such as on vacation, my RPR will rise ten to fourteen points and stay at that elevated level. This obviously is a greater strain on my heart. It takes about one week after a vacation to get the RPR back to my normal range.

I have a digital pulse meter that gives an instant pulse reading. About once a month I take the pulse meter on a jog to see how I am doing. One day while jogging along at about a nine-minute mile pace my pulse rate (PR) stabilized at 135. When I changed from jogging to speed walking, the PR dropped instantly to 110–112. I first thought my pulse meter had malfunctioned. So I tried it several more times on this particular outing and many times since. It repeats and repeats: from jogging to speed walking, 135 PR to 110 PR; from walking to jogging, 110 PR to 135 PR. My breathing would adjust to the pulse rate. I have read that when walking one's legs serve as an auxiliary heart pump. When I really stretched out my stride in speed walking I got the dramatic drops in pulse rate. This tends to support the theory of legs as auxiliary heart pumps.

But now here comes a surprise. Since I started taking chelation therapy, my RPR does not drift to a lower count as a result of sitting still for thirty minutes or longer. Also, my RPR has risen to the fifty-two to fifty-four range and appears to be stable at that point.

Itching

Keeping my food diary helped me isolate the cause of two areas of itching.

The first is on my upper left back in the shoulder blade area. I discovered peanuts have a connection with itching. The more peanuts I ate, the more intense and persistent the itch.

The second is an anus itch. For me this is directly linked to fruit, fresh or otherwise. It is unbelievable how fast this itch starts after a bite of fruit. Oranges seem to trigger it faster than other fruits. If I indulge in too much fruit in too short a period, the anus gets an absolutely raw feeling.

The obvious answer is to watch my diet and not suffer the indignities of having to scratch.

Dry Eyes

Vitamin A cleared up my dry eye problem initially. However, the problem returned.

This time I could generate tears but my eyes still felt dry.

I underwent more food allergy testing, along with some chemical tests. The chemical tests revealed an intolerance to formaldehyde, BHA and BHT. (BHA and BHT are used as preservatives in boxed foods, eg. cereals.)

With some detective work, I determined that my dry eyes were in reality an eye irritation caused by formaldehyde. As you may recall from Chapter 5, most commonly, formaldehyde is used in the manufacturing process of many products. They include:

- plastics—toys, utensils, *eye glasses*
- vinyl, flooring, wallpaper, car interiors
- plywood—formaldehyde is a drying agent for the glue that is used to cement the plies together
- foam rubber—as in pillows and mattresses

I realized formaldehyde caused the irritation to my eyes that imitated the dry eye feeling. I noticed on one of my trips the motel had feather pillows. I got up in the morning without the usual eye irritation. It occurred to me that my foam rubber pillow at home probably contained formaldehyde. The left eye always felt worse than the right probably because I buried the left side of my head in my pillow. Naturally, I replaced the foam rubber pillow at home which resolved this situation.

I also noticed every time I left the house for my early morning jog, the eye irritation disappeared.

The lesson learned here is that dry eyes may be nothing more than persistent eye irritation caused by one's environment. The degree of irritation for me depends on the amount of exposure to formaldehyde. I find instant relief from artificial tears.

Weight Control/Diet

I am here to attest that besides a good diet successful weight control is not achieved without a regular physical exercise program. Also, food allergies and proper digestion often play an important part and should not be overlooked.

Cosmetic Appearance

Proper diet, exercise and rest are a part of the ingredients influencing one's appearance. Also, do not neglect the need for healthy skin. Chelation therapy improves the blood circulation to the skin and elsewhere; and with improved blood circulation, the wrinkles tend to fade. As a side benefit from chelation therapy, many times the age spots disappear or fade significantly, hair color improves, and a sparkle comes to the eyes.

Body Language

The body speaks to us in many different ways and is an accurate indicator of a person's state of wellness. Some of the signs may be well known. The question is do many people *think* and do something to correct the symptoms, or do they ignore the early signs and wait until the situation worsens?

The following list of body language (symptoms) is by no means complete but represents something to think about. These symptoms may mean that your nutritional/health maintenance program needs some adjusting.

- Fingernails
  + white spots indicate a calcium deficiency
  + jagged white lines generally lateral across the fingernail may result from a zinc deficiency
  + brittle nails—calcium and zinc deficiency
- Cold hands and/or feet could mean poor blood circulation; this may well indicate there are circulation problems in other parts of your body. Food allergies are also a causal factor. I was pleased with the warming of my cold hands as the result of the chelation therapy. When I went on the macrobiotic diet I suffered a significant reversal in this regard. A bit of detective work revealed that soybeans, the mainstay of the diet, were the culprit. I knew soybeans were on my food allergy list, but it is from this experience I learned how this particular food allergy manifested itself—
- Nocturnal leg cramps typically result from a calcium deficiency. This may be confused with claudation which is a result of restricted blood flow.

- Pale skin—possible iron deficiency and/or poor circulation.
- Persistent bloating and flatulence—digestive problems suggest malabsorption of nutrients and/or food allergy(ies)
- Persistent foul smelling gas—putrefaction of your food; rotting rather than digestion. This condition strongly suggests a food allergy, and/or problems with the digestive system.

CHAPTER 18

Alternatives for Better Health

This chapter shifts the focus from my personal experience to trying to activate your awareness of alternatives and treatments. The word "awareness" is intended to give you a sense that will make you think, investigate, and make adjustments in your lifestyle. The final word need not be:

- "There is no known cure."
- "You will just have to learn to live with it."
- "You are suffering from a hereditary problem."

Of course, if a person has a bad case of excusitis, all of the above may hold true.

Many people are aware of the standard treatments. However, they fail to realize that many of the treatments only alleviate the symptoms and are not a cure.

This is not a story about us and them—us being the aging population, and them being the medical doctors. Doctors are trained in crisis management with drugs and surgery being their principle approaches. They do wonders with their high-tech equipment for diagnostic aids and treatment. Doctors are interested in scientific double blind studies. They are not interested in anecdotal results. Doctors view such healing occurrences as unique, unexplainable and without scientific evidence to support such anecdotes. However, there is substantial clinical evidence in many areas that lead one to believe that many alternative treatments have validity even though they lack scientific proof.

The mind is a powerful thing, nothing is going to happen until you "make up your mind," and then make it happen. I am sure all of you have conquered some extreme difficulties in the past, but it did not happen until you "made up your mind that you could do it." In this spirit, keep your mind open to the prospect of growing old gracefully can take on a different meaning.

The typical health profile of an aging person may include several of the items below.

- Digestive system distress, increasing bloating and lower bowel gas problems.
- Chest pains occasionally, early symptom of heart disease.
- May be diabetic, having problems with circulation in the legs, and eyesight failing.
- Constipated frequently, and trouble with hemorrhoids.
- On the annual physical, the doctor probably tells a man he has an enlarged prostate; however, this is the accepted norm for an older man (fifty and older)
- Poor colon health, but may be totally unaware.
- Hiatal hernia, proof that you are aging
- Weight problems, have been on many diets but keep ratcheting up and may have totally given up by this time.

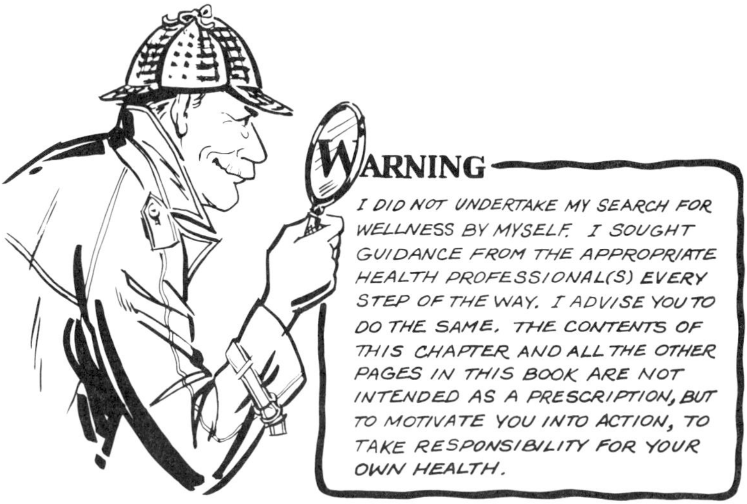

BE YOUR OWN DETECTIVE!

- Maybe not chronic fatigue, but a definite sign the energy level is on the wane.
- Mental alertness diminishing, difficult to concentrate, periods of mental confusion; some early signs of senility showing.
- Dry mouth and dry eyes.
- Hereditary problems.
- Cosmetic appearance unflattering to the ego, dull eyes, complexion losing its healthy look, stiff neck and back, walking at a slower gait.
- Drives a car several times a week—this in itself could alter one's outlook on health in a dramatic way by an accident.

Despite this dreary picture, this man or woman, to the outside world may be aging gracefully—a few aches and pains, yes, but not complaining and accepting one's fate. Most people become resigned and think their problems are here to stay. My contention is it doesn't have to be that way. Some ailments are reversible, and others may be stabilized so they don't get worse; but, nothing is going to happen until you "make up your mind" and make some changes.

It is beneficial to acknowledge that the body is a chemical factory. If there is a dysfunction, there is a reason for it; it does not "just happen." However, the underlying cause is often elusive. Many times a cure, as opposed to treating the symptom, may not be readily apparent.

The body has tremendous capabilities to cure itself. On the other hand, it can take heavy abuse and can keep on functioning for years—maybe not at an optimum level, but it does keep going. A healthy body needs some cooperation on our part. Once you start to think about the body language and react to it, improvements in your health can be realized.

I would like to address the ailments detailed above to give you an awareness about health maintenance and some alternatives to consider. I have focused on this subject for the past six years and believe there should be a new meaning given to growing old gracefully and not suffering in silence. In my own case I overcame eleven items, listed above and some not listed (I am not a diabetic). The pay-off for me is:

- increased energy level
- mental alertness restored
- flattering cosmetic changes; all is vanity!
- improved cardiovascular function

DIGESTIVE SYSTEM DISTRESS

This situation can take on different characteristics—the extreme being ulcers or colitis. But let me just talk about bloating and lower bowel gas. This typically comes on after eating and it is a body's signal telling you something is not right. But are you listening? When we bloat badly, sometimes we say "It must have been something I ate." That is probably true. But if this happens time after time, day after day, you are doing something wrong. Think about it!

The cause of bloating and gas are commonly one or a combination of those things listed below:

- Eating too fast—gulping your food down. You need to realize chewing generates enzymes in your mouth necessary to the digestive process. If you gulp your food down too fast, you don't get enough enzymes into the food, so consequently the chemical reaction when the food gets to your stomach is poor. If you do not believe this, put it to a test and stand by for a case of indigestion.
- Drinking a lot of liquids while eating dilutes the digestive juices. As you age, the digestive juices do not flow as freely as they did in younger years. You should eat your food without washing it down.
- Food combinations—different foods require different enzymes and times to be digested. When you combine incompatible foods, here comes another episode of a stomach upset. Some of these food combinations may be a great surprise to you—they surprised me. Think about the American diet versus some of the food-combining rules:
- fruit should be eaten by itself, on an empty stomach.
- Proteins and starches are incompatible.
- Beef and potatoes do not mix.

  And the list goes on. In my personal case, my digestive system is less than par and when I fail to observe some of these food combining rules, I get indigestion. Since I do not care for this type of distress, I have had to change my eating habits. The health food store abounds with information about the do's and don't's of food combining, including charts to put up on your kitchen wall. The art of food combining is a subject I recommend for those in search of better health.

- The bloating can be a result of the lack of action on the part of your pancreas. Different times during the digestive process, it is supposed to furnish enzymes to aid that process. However, if it fails to provide the enzymes after you are through eating, within about five minutes the bloating will start. I found by one or two Pancreatin Enzyme tablets after eating, the bloating does not occur. Consequently, I do not have to take an antacid remedy which relieves the bloating, but leeches out vitamin C.
- You are certainly mindful of some foods which may give you a problem. The symptoms from these "food allergies" may not reveal themselves as rashes or runny eyes or dripping sinus. They may manifest themselves in other ways. But food allergies should not be ruled out as a probable cause of repeated digestive distress. There are books on the market that can help you to understand the food allergy problem. I will list those later in the bibliograpy of recommended reading.

CHEST PAINS

If you are having chest pains occasionally, do you think about this as a signal calling for corrective action? Of course, it could be gas, but you may assume it is "approaching old age." Your body is telling you something is wrong. You have a circulatory problem.

As the chest pains worsen, the eventuality is the crisis treatment of bypass surgery. Bypass surgery is not a cure, it only treats the symptom. If you do not change your living habits, you will be back for a second bypass. There are alternatives to bypass surgery.

• Nathan Pritikin, the author of *Program of Diet and Exercise* reversed his condition strictly by a nutrition and exercise approach. Other people who have followed his program of diet and exercise have achieved similar success.

• There is a protocol called "chelation therapy" that is not generally accepted by the American Medical Association establishment. However, it is approved by the Federal Drug Administration. It is a legitimate alternative to bypass surgery. Chelation therapy is the intravenous feeding of a chemical called "ethylene-diamine-tetra-acetate—EDTA." The original application of this therapy was for lead poisoning. Intravenous administration of EDTA chelated (latched on to) the toxic lead and eliminated it from the body through the normal elimination process, through the kidneys. Some years back, several factory workers came down with lead poisoning. As a consequence, they were given chelation therapy. The doctors noted that besides eliminating the lead and restoring the person to health, many other remarkable improvements were noted. One of the improvements observed was the opening up the arteries of heart patients, allowing a better cardiovascular function.

Early on, experimentation with the strength of the dose and the time of feeding resulted in some kidney failures. The failures were attributed to overdosing the kidneys from two standpoints:

- giving the patient too strong a dose in too short a time; and/or
- treating patients with weak kidneys who can't stand a normal dose.

In time, a new medical association established a protocol for the safe administration of EDTA. The protocol requires a thorough examination prior to treatment so the doctor has a good understanding of the health of the kidneys, and the strength of the dosage to be specified. Since that time, for all of those doctors who observed the protocol, they do not have one known death from the treatment of chelation therapy. This compares with heart bypass surgery that results in three to five percent mortality rate (depending on source) from the operation.

I am aware of an article in a respected magazine that says chelation therapy is not effective. The author probably never talked to the people who have availed themselves of this treatment; nor does he seem aware of the mass of clinical records supporting the efficacy of this treatment. If he were, he would have quite a different story to tell. Patients who use chelation therapy come close to being cured and return to an active life. They do not become heart cripples as so often is the case with bypass surgery.

I recently heard (Nov. 1989) a respected doctor on his talk show acknowledge that he has many letters from people attesting to the goodness of chelation therapy. His response to this is there is no scientific proof and if this were a valid treatment protocol you would see doctors taking the treatment. He summarily rejected chelation therapy because the only support it had was anecdotal information.

When I heard this, I reflected on my own experience. It was that very week that I sat in a treatment room with six other people. Among them were three of special interest:

- An 82 year old chemist PhD. who had two quadruple bypasses. He needed a third but his health was so poor he would not survive the operation. Chelation therapy was his salvation. He is no longer a heart cripple—out and active.

- A pharmacist, about age 70 with a bypass that failed. He, too, was realizing the excellent results from chelation therapy in restoring his health.
- The third individual, a retired educator possessing a doctorate degree. His story the same, a failed bypass, and returned to health by chelation therapy.

The above anecdotal accounts are in reality a part of the chelation therapy clinical record being amassed. I am sure you would be convinced of the efficacy of this treatment if you would visit the doctor's clinic that provides this service and talk with the patients.

The American College for the Advancement in Medicine (ACAM), (714) 583–7666, can give you the name of a doctor in your area who provides chelation therapy. (You may be surprised to know that many medical doctors are not even aware of this treatment.)

FOR THE DIABETIC PERSON:

Heart disease many times slowly evolves into diminished circulation in the legs and, in some cases, the eyesight begins to fail at a rapid pace.

The lack of circulation often results in leg and foot ulcers. Many times these ulcers become very large—three to four inches in diameter, down to the raw muscle, runny and ugly. It does not respond to antibiotic treatment, either externally or internally. This situation continues to degenerate until gangrene is in evidence. This is the time surgical intervention becomes the prescribed treatment. Of course, for some, they may first try surgical techniques to open up the arteries in the legs; but in so many cases amputation becomes inevitable.

Diabetics often have failing eyesight, it fails rapidly as the circulation in the eyeball diminishes.

An abundance of clinical records (anecdotes) show treatment with EDTA as described above restores the circulation sufficiently to cure the leg and foot ulcers and return the eyesight back to normal. This has to be one of the best kept secrets in the world.

As you investigate this, the government and many doctors will tell you not to trust any one thing that cures everything. But let me present this: aspirin is taken for headaches, pains or colds; in all these cases, it is working on the neurological system—doing something to alleviate pain. In the case of chelation therapy it improves the cardiovascular function and the flow of blood has to do with the entire body. Consequently, if the body is being better nourished, whatever body function is hurting, it is going to come back closer to a state of wellness. Think about it!

CONSTIPATION AND HEMORRHOIDS

This situation is most unpleasant. I suffered from this for years; first with the constipation, and the continued straining that brought on the hemorrhoids.

I'm sure many of you also have suffered for years. There are all kinds of hype advertising this, that and the other; more bulk, more whatever, and yes, constipation is very directly diet-related. If you are constipated, you are doing something wrong.

Nutrition experts agree that the digestive system needs fiber, but people generally do not know that meat provides no fiber, and bread provides very little. Artificial bulk may provide temporary help, but it does not correct the underlying problem. Another cause of constipation may be traced to a food allergy. Food allergies manifest themselves in many different ways.

The digestive system which works like a chemical factory has an approximate four-day cycle, from start to finish. Whatever one may eat today will have an immediate effect, and whatever effect, good or bad, it will begin diminishing over a four-day period. Keeping a diet diary helps to isolate offending foods for constipation or other kinds of ailments. When the constipation is gone, the hemorrhoids inevitably disappear.

PROSTATE

Statistics reveal that about 70% of the men, by the time they reach the age of 65, will have had prostate problems. Out of this, a high number of people experience cancer—some of them caught early enough, some of them not. The University of Texas Lifetime Health Letter, October 1989, indicates that 400,000 to 500,000 operations are done each year to surgically shave away the prostate growth that causes obstruction and interferes with urination.

The male reproductive organs are a major storehouse for zinc. When you have an orgasm, there is a loss of zinc. When it depletes to a certain point, prostate problems begin; it is most common for it to enlarge. The enlargement eventually begins to choke off the urinary tract. Dr. Michael A. Weiner, in *Nutrition Against Aging,* Chapter 7 addresses the difficulties with prostate health. He states (page 116) that the proper amount of zinc intake will prevent the prostate trouble typically experienced by men in their fifties and sixties.

I suffered for twenty years with a prostate problem, antibiotics did not work. To me, the bottom line is to take the RDA zinc as a preventive measure. Zinc therapy will relieve prostatitis. Fourteen years ago I made that discovery. On a more recent physical examination for the prostate, the doctor said "This is very strange." I said, "What is strange?" He replied, "You have a prostate the size I would expect to find in a young man. I have never seen this before in a man of your age (65 years old)."

COLON HEALTH

Many people come down with diverticulitis or colitis. In both cases, it involves inflammation of the colon or large intestine. Colon health is connected to constipation and it is connected to our diet. Many times you will say "I've got a constipation headache." No doubt, you are right, and when you're relieved, the headache goes away. You may be surprised to know the colon is connected to many other parts of the body. Constipation is one way to clog up your system. Just because you got rid of your constipation headache, does not necessarily mean you are cleaned out.

Years and years of eating mucus-forming foods such as bread and milk leads to a condition where the mucus becomes impacted in the folds and on the walls of the colon. This interferes with the peristaltic action necessary in the elimination process. When this happens, you have a colon in less than robust health and susceptible to disease. The disease of cancer is all too prevalent. I question whether cancer would ever happen in a clean, healthy colon.

To me, it seems prudent to have colon irrigation for an accurate determination of its state of cleanliness. If it proves to need the colonic therapy, two things should be considered:

- alter your diet to avoid mucus-forming foods
- repeat the colonic therapy about twice a year

Milk is absolutely dynamite to many people who have a lactose intolerance of the colon. The pain can become intense. Being knowledgeable of this and adjusting your diet may save you from developing colitis or diverticulitis. Since becoming informed, I have not had a return bout of diverticulitis; however, I had suffered with great pain in four episodes.

HIATAL HERNIA

This situation develops because a part of the stomach works its way above the diaphragm muscle. Generally, the advice will be to elevate the head of your bed to make it more tolerable for sleeping; and "learn to live with it."

It is highly probable this condition develops because of a sedentary life. Many people habitually lie down for a nap or go to bed before the food eaten has a chance to digest. Many doctors recommend not lying down until at least two hours after eating. The stomach pulsates as it prepares the food you swallowed to be passed on to the small intestine in the digestive process. It is believed this action leads to pushing the stomach through the diaphragm to cause the hiatal hernia.

If you already suffer from a hiatal hernia there may be a chance for correction. I know of one health professional who suggests the following technique:

- Drink a large glass of water (12 ounces)
- Exercise on a rebounder (small trampoline) for ten minutes twice a day
- Repeat the above process until the hernia corrects itself.

This action should slowly shake down the stomach to where it belongs.

Hiatal hernias do not "just happen."

WEIGHT PROBLEMS

Everybody seems to know about weight problems, the many diets available and how typically most people, rather than keeping the weight down, ratchet up. After a few years they wind up being too heavy and miserable.

Documented evidence indicates food allergies are many times the cause of being unable to lose weight. One case comes to mind: a friend, a thirty-five year-old, 240-pound woman, five feet four inches tall. I suggested to her food allergy(s) may be the underlying cause of her excessive weight. By taking the pulse test, discussed earlier in Chapter 5, she found wheat to be the culprit. She altered her diet to eliminate wheat and wheat products and lost twelve pounds the first week.

This is not to suggest that if you stop eating wheat the same thing will happen to you. But it does suggest that if you become a diet detective and start a food elimination program, you will discover the foods causing the weight gain. It is apparent that food allergies, in many cases, cause a dysfunction in a person's basic metabolism.

Aside from diet, to be successful at controlling weight, regular exercise is necessary. Once you get into the habit, it is not such a chore. In my case, with a 5'11" frame, my weight edged up over the years to 200 pounds; not excessively overweight in my mind but a long way from the desired weight.

After getting an understanding of my food allergies, my weight is now 155, trim, and slim and happy about it. However, I did not achieve lasting success until regular exercise became a part of my regimen.

FATIGUE—THAT TIRED FEELING

When one has a tired feeling, it is often vague, seemingly unexplainable and it is generally accepted as a part of getting old. This is about as far from the truth as can be. You certainly are aware of how important diet and exercise is to your general health and well-being; and that affects your energy level as well.

But let me pose something you may not think about—the power of the brain and why you need exercise.

Are you aware that your brain is in control of your body? This may sound like a stupid statement, but remember your muscles and bones respond to your brain. When the brain says, "I am tired," you get an instant response from your muscles and bones, "indeed your are tired." Do you say to yourself, "Boy, am I tired. I didn't sleep at all well last night." Does it become ritual day after day? After you get busy and stop thinking tired, things go well until the middle of the afternoon (3:00–4:00 P.M.). It's getting toward the end of the work day and it is time to feel tired; the afternoon fade. The question is, do you program yourself to be tired?

To help deprogram yourself to stop thinking tired, play a little game. You might call it a liar's game, because it may not always be the truth. When anybody asks "how are you?" respond with "super great," "magnificient," or "outstanding" as though you mean it. After saying that about fifteen or twenty times by the end of the day, you *will* feel super great, not tired. "Make up you mind" that you are not going to be tired until you get to bed. Over time you will achieve success and not "think tired" anymore.

This approach may seem unusual or difficult to grasp, but the positive results I experienced makes me believe it will work for anyone who accepts the challenge to try it.

You recall in an earlier chapter, I presented the body elimination functions. The one I want to heighten your awareness of is the lymphatic system. Remember, it does not have its own pump, but depends on muscle movement to a great extent.

The lymphatic system not only carries off toxins, it nourishes the body. It is essential to the basic metabolism in the digestive process. Consequently, if the lymphatic system is sluggish, a tired and rundown feeling is sure to ensue.

There are lymph nodes in the front and back of your chest; in the groin area and elsewhere. When taking brisk walks, many health books advise you to "swing the arms." When jogging, exaggerate the twisting of the torso to help the lymphatic system eliminate the toxic buildup, and promote the basic metabolism.

I have a difference of opinion on the subject of exercise. Many books say three times a week as minimum; some recommend five times a week. I believe you should exercise every day to keep the lymphatic system working. After all, do you want it to go on vacation just because you don't exercise?

DIMINISHING MENTAL ALERTNESS

This situation takes on different characteristics such as difficulty in concentrating, inability to express oneself, or mental confusion. Most people accept this as the normal aging process. To the public this is the early signs of senility starting to show. The awareness of potential underlying causes, other than aging, is obscure. Two elements bear investigation and understanding.

One aspect can be from your teeth. Many people have cavities. And most people have their cavities filled with mercury amalgam, but they do not realize mercury is a deadly poison to the body. Not just your body or my body, but everybody's body. The dental profession instruction is not to touch this with their bare hands; but it is all right to put in your mouth, a contradiction I don't understand. They hasten to say that if it is handled carefully and after it is stabilized there is no danger. That is not the case. Remember, your body is a chemical factory and when some other chemicals come in contact with mercury, there is a reaction. And with certain chemicals you can have a deadly reaction. The mercury by itself might interface with your neurological system and can be the cause of some tragic results, including behavior symptomatic of approaching senility. It is suggested that you proceed with a hair test to determine toxic mineral levels.

Many people are not aware of another toxic metal, aluminum. If you have an excess of this, it could impact your neurological system and there's no telling what body part(s) or function(s) may be affected. They have found in some cases that excess aluminum is a factor in Alzheimer's patients.

Chelation therapy eliminates the toxic metals—aluminum, mercury, lead and others—from your body. Significant clinical records substantiate this assertion. Some of the books providing greater detail on this subject are identified at the end of this chapter.

DRY EYES AND MOUTH

Many older people are troubled with this condition. The dry mouth and the dry eyes started me out to find relief when my family doctor told me "there is no known cure." I found he was probably correct—no known *drug* cure. However, I did find that vitamin supplementation greatly alleviated the dry mouth and eyes. Vitamins A and C did wonders, (not mega doses) so I did not have to take artificial saliva for my mouth and artificial tears for my eyes. However, my mouth tended to dryness occasionally but still without need of supplementation of artificial saliva.

I did find that MSG (monosodium glutamate), the flavor enhancer, turns my mouth dry, quickly, so I try to avoid MSG (Chinese restaurant favorite).

Unexpectedly, I found the final cure to be in the bite of my mouth. As strange as it may seem, an adjustment in my bite did the trick (as discussed in Chapter 16).

HEREDITY

It may be true because of your heritage you may have the genes that make you more vulnerable to certain diseases. However, in my opinion, this rationale is overworked in many cases. The probabilities are this happens because the same health habits are adopted by the succeeding generation. The tendency to be overweight or to have heart attacks can be overcome by change in diet and exercise patterns. Examine your situation before you accept that "it runs in the family" look for alternative lifestyles to break the chain.

COSMETIC CHANGES

A change in living habits dramatically alters a person's physical appearance. In my search for wellness the following cosmetic changes are in evidence.

- my teeth turned from ivory yellow to white
- 155 pounds looks a lot better than 200 pounds on a 5'11" frame.
- eyes from dull to a super sparkle
- no more dandruff, talk about a shampoo lasting for three days. I have not seen any dandruff in more than six years!
- the onset of the typical gray pallor of my complexion changed to a more healthy look and feel.

AUTOMOBILE SAFETY

The popular slogan is "drive defensively." I'm not sure what this is supposed to mean, but it seems to say: "The other guy is nuts and I am the only one who knows how to drive safely." A far better slogan would be, "*Think smart* and *drive smart*." "See and be seen." To see means to know—it means to think. Three cases are given to illustrate the point.

- At dawn and dusk, and during the day, in conditions of some reduced visibility, you may habitually drive with your lights off, or with the parking lights on. Because you can see to drive without the headlights, you want to save the battery. Have you ever considered though *you* can see well enough to drive, the approaching driver may not see you without your headlights? You should *be aware* that without headlights under these conditions, you are difficult to see, and what someone does not see might be the reason for so many accidents. The Greyhound Bus Company some years ago adopted a policy to drive with their headlights on all the time. When they first started doing this, their accident rate decreased something like 6%. The Chesapeake Bay Bridge Tunnel toll gate person asks drivers to "turn on your headlights for safety" during daylight hours. Think about that!

- You're driving down a throughfare, and have the right of way and you see somebody coming out of a driveway—not backing out, but driving straight out—but there are some telephone poles and bushes. Do you see that his vision is obscured and that he probably does not see you and may pull right out in front of you as you progress down the street? To see is to think and to know.
- You're driving down a multi-lane street, and as you are overtaking a car whether you are on the left or right side of him, there is a blind area in his rear view mirror. You should be mindful of this. His actions may appear to be erratic. He might pull over right in front of you because he does not see you. Another blind man is one with fogged up or frosted windows. His actions may also seem erratic to you. But as you see and think and are *aware,* you will be prepared and give the lead driver warning you are overtaking him. Be wary of his blind area.

The foregoing should make you more safety conscious, so you are going to live longer.

SUMMARY

The list of things I talked about are not all inclusive, but are only a sample of alternative treatments. I believe many of these may be better than what is being presented to you. But guaranteed, nothing will change until "make up your mind." Nothing is going to happen until you expend the effort to make it happen. Be all you can be!

REFERENCES

Listed here are some of the recommended sources of information to help you prepare for your "health attack." Most of these references contain anecdotal information to prove their point.

- *Food is Your Best Medicine,* by Dr. Henry Beiler, M.D.; publisher Ballantine Books. (This will give you a good understanding of the body functions as a chemical factory.)
- *Pritikin Program of Diet and Exercise,* by Nathan Pritikin; publisher Grosset and Dunlop. (The Pritikin Program has met with great success in controlling high blood pressure, and improving the cardiovascular function to avoid the need for bypass surgery.)
- *Pass or Bypass? Chelation Extends Life,* by Dr. James J. Julian; publisher Wellness Press. (Details on chelation therapy are presented.)
- *Bypassing Bypass,* by Dr. Elmer Cranton, M.D. and Arlene Brecher; Stein and Day publisher. (Explains chelation therapy and the goodness of it beyond the treatment for heart disease. Chapter 7 identifies several other health problems overcome by improvement of the cardiovascular function.)
- *Nutrition Against Aging,* by Michael A. Weiner, PhD. and Kathleen Goss; Publisher Bantam Books. (This work addresses many of the "aging diseases" from a nutritional standpoint. My experience agrees with what he presents.)
- *It's All in Your Head,* by Dr. Hal A. Huggins, D.D.S., and S. A. Huggins, R.D.H., P. O. Box 2589, Colorado

Springs, CO 80901. (This presents in detail the devastating effects of mercury amalgam.)

- *Chiropractic in New Zealand; Report by Commission of Inquiry,* P. D. Hasselberg, Government Printer. (This work is a classic. If you have had any doubts about the efficacy of chiropractic treatment, this should dispel those doubts. The testimony from medical doctors to counter the chiropractic community failed to discredit the usefulness of chiropractic care.)
- *Colon Health,* by Dr. Norman W. Walker, D.Sc. PhD.; Publisher, Norwalk Press. (Reading this work will make you aware of the need to pay attention to colon health.)
- *The Complete Book of Vitamins.* Rodale Press. (If you take vitamins, this is a good reference to keep you from going astray.)
- *Prescription Drugs' Side Effects Revealed,* by Gayle Cawood, et. al. (If you are taking prescription drugs, this will give you the details on the side effects)
- *The Allergy Self Help Book,* by Sharon Faelten and the editors of Prevention Magazine; Publisher, Rodale Press. (Don't overlook the need to keep a diet diary and follow the guidelines to identify your allergies. Once found and eliminated, guaranteed you will be pleased with the change.)

EPILOGUE

This is the end of the book, but this is not the end of my story. As I write this I am 66 years old. I have been on my *search for wellness* for more than six years. I continue to strive for the understanding of various therapies in the treatment of health problems.

There is no panacea for maintaining your health. Diet and exercise are a good beginning. By continued research and playing detective (mostly, keeping a diet diary and recording how I felt physically from day to day) I made some astonishing discoveries.

With the help and guidance of health professionals—medical doctor, dentist, chiropractor, dietitian/nutritionist, I am happy with the progress I have made in my search for wellness. I believe I have set my biological clock back at least fifteen years, and have slowed the aging process.

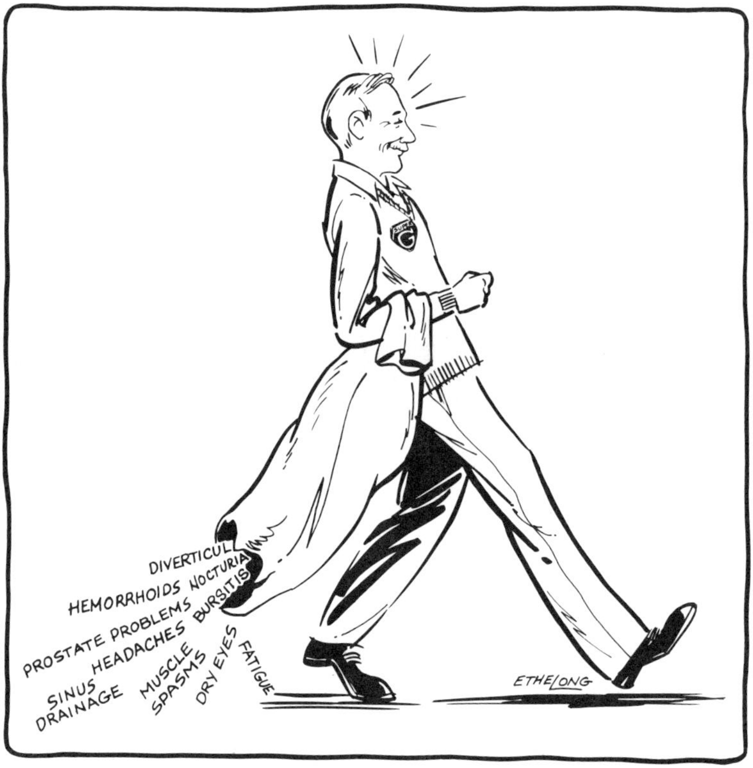

I continue to be guided and encouraged by the old saying "Ask, and it shall be given you. Seek, and ye shall find. Knock, and it shall be opened unto you. For everyone who asketh, receiveth; and he that seeketh, findeth; and to him that knocketh it shall be opened." Matthew 7:7,8

I trust you, the reader, have benefited from reading this book. I hope your curiosity has been aroused and that you are ready to assume responsibility for your own health. The Army exhorts its men and women to "be all you can be." If you don't like what you see, nothing is going to happen until you make some changes. The starting point of maintaining your health begins with you. Make your life an adventure to be enjoyed!

Appendix A

Special permission was granted to use extracts and/or quotations from the following references.

1. *It's All in Your Head,* by Dr. Hal A. Huggins, D.D.S. and S. A. Huggins, R.D.H., c. 1985. p 58–62
2. *Chiropractic in New Zealand;* Report by Commission of Inquiry, P. D. Hasselburg, Government Printer, Wellington, New Zealand. (Reprinted by Palmer College of Chiropractic, Davenport, Iowa by special permission.) p 72–79
3. *Pass or Bypass? Chelation Extends Life,* by Dr. James J. Julian, M.D.; publisher Wellness Press, 1654 Cahuenga Blvd., Hollywood, CA 90028, c. 1981. p 87–89
4. *Homogenized!,* by Nicholas Sampsidis, M.S., Sunflower Publishing, Inc., Glenwood Landing, NY 11547, c. 1983. p 120–121
5. *Mineral Analysis Report,* Doctor's Data, P. O. Box 111, 30 W 101 Roosevelt Road, West Chicago, IL 60185. p 100–107
6. Pamphlet *Get the Big Picture About Health,* distributed by Dr. John H. Gerath, Jane Lew, West Virginia (author not indicated). p 116

7. *Thermagraphic Analysis* and brochures by Therma-Scan, Inc., 21519 Harper, St. Clair Shores, MI 48080. p 117–120

8. *Hippocrates Health Institute,* Brian R. Clement, Director, 1443 Palmdale Court, West Palm Beach, FL 33411. p 131–132, 137–139, 149, 197–200

Appendix B

REFERENCES

Men's Health, Rodale Press, 33 E. Minor Street, Emmaus, PA 18049. (Subscription, 1 year—$24)

Gary Null's Natural Living Newsletter, NLN Publications, P. O. Box 849, Madison Square Station, New York, NY 10010. (Subscription 12 issues, 1 year—$28.00)

University of California, Berkeley Wellness Letter, P. O. Box 10922, Des Moines, Iowa 50340. (Subscription 12 issues, 1 year—$18.00)

American Institute for Cancer Research Newsletter. 1759 R Street N.W., Washington, DC 20009 (non-profit organization)

Mayo Clinic Health Letter, Mayo Medical Resources, Rochester, MN 55905 (Subscription, 1 year—$24.00)

Nutrition Action Health Letter. Center for Science in the Public Interest, 1501 16th Street N.W., Washington DC 20036 (annual dues—$19.95; special rates for seniors—$14.95)

Food is Your Best Medicine, by Dr. Henry Bieler, M.D., Publisher Ballantine Books, 201 E. 50th Street, New York, NY 10022, c. 1984 (fourth printing).

Pritikin Program for Diet and Exercise, by Nathan Pritikin, publisher Grosset and Dunlap, c. 1979.

Pass or Bypass? Chelation Extends Life, by Dr. James J. Julian, M.D.; publisher Wellness Press, 1654 Cahuenga Blvd., Hollywood, CA 90028, c. 1981.

Bypassing Bypass, by Dr. Elmer Cranton, M.D. and Arlene Brecher; Stein and Day Publisher, c. 1984.

Nutrition Against Aging by Michael A. Weiner, PhD. and Kathleen Goss; Bantam Books publisher, New York, c. 1983.

The Pulse Test, Easy Allergy Detection, by Dr. Arthur F. Coca, M.D.; ARCO Publishing, Inc., 219 Park Ave. South, New York, NY 10003.

It's All in Your Head, by Dr. Hal A. Huggins, D.D.S. and S. A. Huggins, R.D.H., c. 1985.

Chiropractic in New Zealand; Report by Commission of Inquiry, P. D. Hasselburg, Government Printer, Wellington, New Zealand. (Reprinted by Palmer College of Chiropractic, Davenport, Iowa by special permission.)

Recalled by Life, by Anthony J. Sattilaro, M.D., Publisher Avon Books, 105 Madison Ave., NY 10016.

Nutrition Against Disease by Dr. Roger J. Williams, Bantam Books published by arrangement with Pitman Publishing Corp., 6 East 43rd St., New York, NY 10017

Appendix C

HIPPOCRATES LIVING FOOD RECIPES

Carrot-Spinach Juice

3 cups carrot juice
1 bunch spinach (1/2 pound)
1/4 yellow bell pepper
1/4 red bell pepper
1/4 avocado
1 ounce liquid amino
1 tsp. brown celergy seed powder
1 small fresh blinder
Blend in the blender.

Bell Pepper Stuffed (for four people)

+ 4 ounces oyster mushroom or shitaki mushroom or artichoke hearts. Slice thin with a knife.
+ 1/4 of small onion, minced with a knife
+ 1/2 cauliflower, shredded in food processor
+ 1/2 cup, 1/4 pound sesame tehene butter in food processor with S blade

+ 2 stalks of celery in processor with juice of one lemon
+ 1 tbsp. of chili powder
+ 2 tbsp. fresh oregano leaves
+ 2 ounces liquid amino

Mix in all ingredients and stuff.

Cauliflower (substitute for rice)

1 head cauliflower, shredded in processor
1/2 red, 1 1/2 yellow pepper, chopped
1/2 bunch of fresh mint leaves, minced
add liquid amino

Sauce (in blender)

1/2 cup sesame tehene
1 ounce liquid amino
1/2 of lemon juice
1/4 cup water

Blended to a mayonnaise-like consistency. Then mix ingredients

Apple Pie with Fig Nut Crust

Crust:

10 dried Calmyra figs
2 cups shelled almonds or filberts
1 tbsp. powdered psyllium husks
Distilled water

Soak figs and nuts overnight in distilled water. Soaking the nuts removes the enzyme inhibitor that is present on the skin of all nuts and seeds. The moisture absorbed by the nuts makes them more digestible. Insert "S" blade into your food processor and add the drained nuts and figs. Grind both ingredients into a thick dough. If too thick, add a tbsp. or two of water, or only enough to make it a stiff consistency. Sprinkle powdered psyllium husks over the top and mix again in processor. Press the dough into a 9″ pyrex pie plate and dry in a dehydrator for 2 hours. If you don't have a dehydrator, turn your oven onto the lowest temperature possible and allow the crust to dry in the oven from 30 minutes to one hour. It should feel dry to the touch, so test frequently and make a notation of time required for future use.

Filling:

3 Delicious apples
1 banana
1/2 cup fine shredded coconut
3/4 cup raisins, soaked 1/2 hour
1/2 tsp. cinnamon
1/4 tsp. nutmeg
1/4 cup almond butter or tahini
1 tbsp. powdered psyllium husks
juice of 1/2 lemon

Peel the apples, cut into quarters and remove seeds. Allow them to soak in enough water to cover. Add lemon juice to prevent browning. In a bowl, add the soaked and drained raisins, the shredded coconut, the almond butter or tahini, and the cinnamon and nutmeg and mix thoroughly. Place the drained apples into your food processor with the "S" blade in place and add the banana cut into 1″ pieces. Add the raisin coconut mixture and process thoroughly. Sprinkle the psyllium husks over the top and mix again. If the mixture does not move in the processor, add tiny amounts of water. The consistency should be that of a thick pudding. Fill the crust and decorate with any seasonal fruits or nuts. Refrigerate. Serves 6–8.

NOTE: Most of these ingredients are available in health food stores. Psyllium husks are an excellent source of dietary fiber and work like gelatin to keep the filling firm. A dehydrator is an important piece of equipment for people following a living food diet. You can make a large variety of delicious desserts and snacks that are nourishing, as well.

Vegetable Sushi

$1\frac{1}{2}$ cups raw pumpkin seeds
$1\frac{1}{2}$ cups shelled raw almonds
1 large stalk of broccoli
1 red bell pepper, minced
2 or 3 large garlic cloves, minced
1 onion, minced
$\frac{1}{8}$ cup Braggs Liquid Aminos
Nori sheets (seaweed)
Alfalfa sprouts

Soak the pumpkin seeds and almonds overnight in distilled water. Drain and place them in your blender. Run the broccoli through your Champion juicer using the homogenizing insert. Add the minced pepper, garlic and onion and mix together. Pour the Liquid Aminos into the blender and add the broccoli mixture. Blend all these ingredients until smooth.

Place a nori sheet on a smooth surface, and using a pastry brush or your fingers, moisten it with distilled water. Cover the sheet with some of the alfalfa sprouts and place spoonfuls of the seed/nut mixture in a row about 1″ from the edge of the sheet. Make the mixture about $1\frac{1}{2}$″ in diameter, about like a sausage. Carefully roll up the nori sheet and cut into $2\frac{1}{2}$ or 3″ lengths. Follow same procedure with remaining sheets. Arrange the sushi around your salad platter. This is a delicious finger food and so good for you. Serves 6–8 people.

NOTE: Braggs is a concentrated liquid protein made from soybeans. It contains no sodium and is used as a seasoning to replace salt. It can be purchased at most health food stores.

INDEX